Vol. I

~ Written and Produced by:
Dhurva Lama

~ Clinically approved and recommended by:

University/Salk Institute Scientist
Jamie Whyte MD

~ Dhurva® Models:

**Stephania Ochs
Sofie Blicher
Shelby Lawson
Yoshi M.
Dhurva Lama**

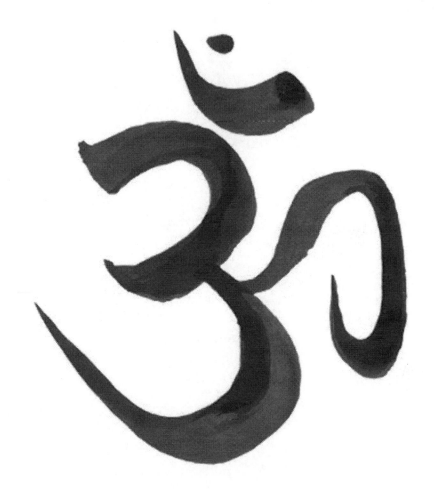

II

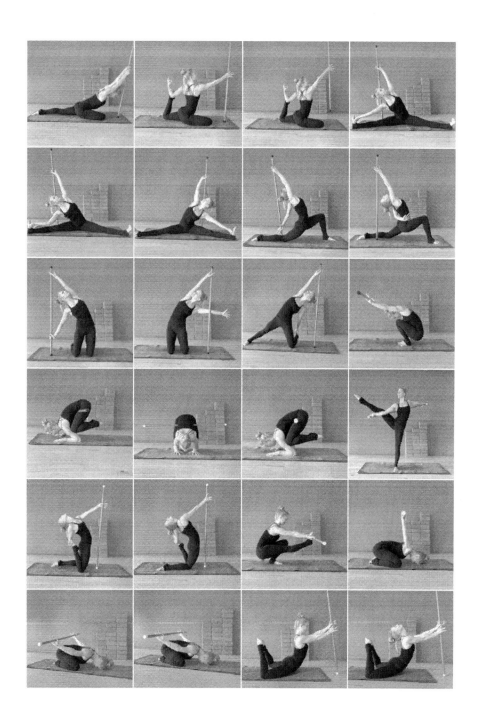

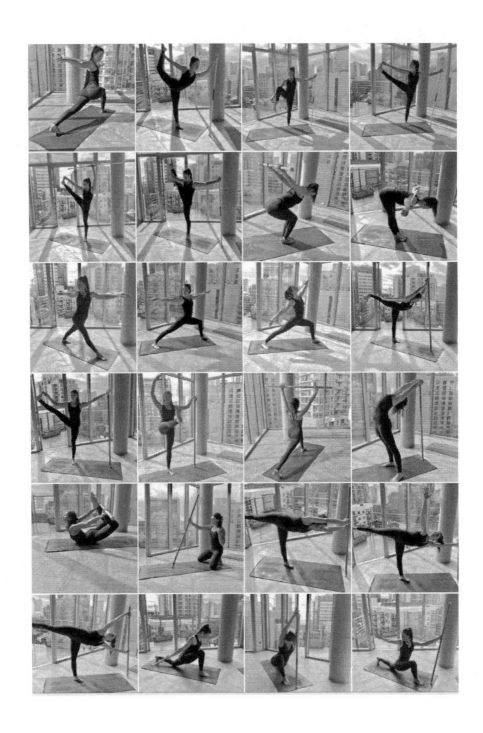

IV

Jamie Whyte - *Physician*

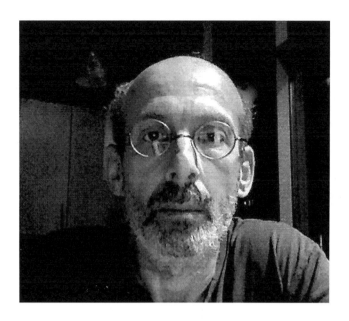

-BIOGRAPHY-

Dr. Whyte began his professional life in industry, working for his family's manufacturing concern. After the business was sold he took up the study of medicine, ultimately earning his M.D. and becoming a Director of the Sleep Disorders Center at Columbia-Presbyterian Medical Center in New York City. After several years of professional practice he pursued an interest in law, obtaining a J.D. degree via the Law, Science and Technology program at Arizona State University.

Then it was a move further west and back to science after being awarded a microbiology fellowship at the Salk Institute in La Jolla, California. There, Dr. Whyte conducted research on the interactions among exercise, metabolism and aging. Now on his fourth career, Dr. Whyte is currently a writer and entrepreneur based in San Diego

-YOGA AND FITNESS PHILOSOPHY-

In fitness, as elsewhere, balance and harmony are the essentials. And in this regard yoga is unique among all forms of physical activity. The yogic philosophy acknowledges excellence but this recognition is aspirational, not competitive. It is uninhibited in its appreciation of the human form while avoiding the destructive obsession with physical appearance. A thoughtful practice almost magically integrates and harmonizes physicalism with spiritualism. Modern yoga expresses the wisdom of millennia yet still remains an openness to new forms and new ideas. If not a perfect system of exercise, yoga is the closest thing that we mortals have thus far devised.

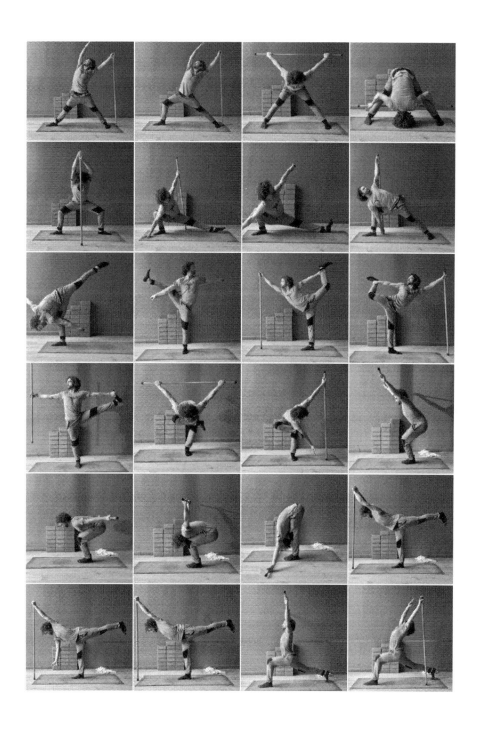

Dominic Mineo - *Author*

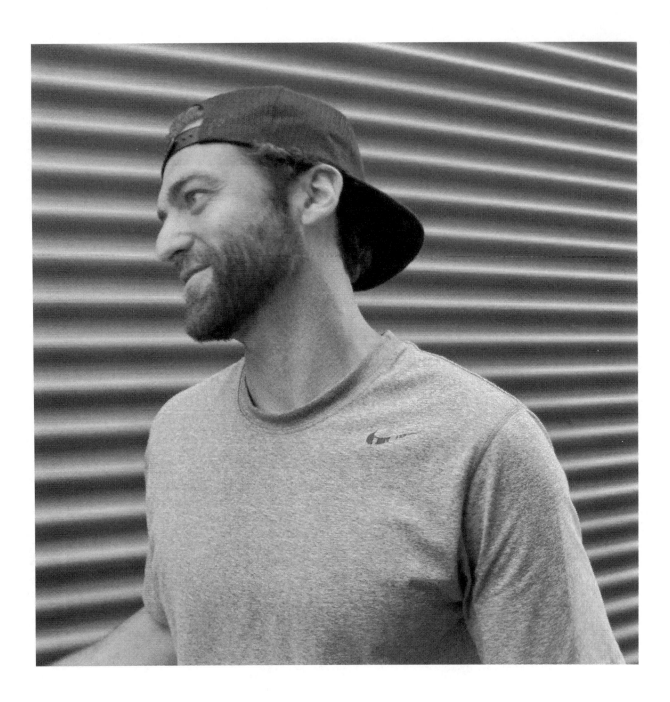

VIII

-BIOGRAPHY-

My interest in natural healing and caring for my body brought me to Yoga. Fascinated by the unique physical challenge and sudden mental clarity from self awareness, I enrolled in a teacher training program.
I spent the next the next 8 years teaching and practicing in over 50 countries and all seven continents. Time forward, I'm now broadcasting the Dhurva Yoga® brand across the globe making body therapy a necessity for self-care.

-YOGA AND FITNESS PHILOSOPHY-

I personally practice and teach functional movement Yoga. These movements induce a strong, flexible base through gymnastic core strength using articulate hand and foot balance.
Meditation, calmness and practicing patience promote a healing relaxed state which enables focus and attention span to grow. Meditation also makes you aware, that your inner attitude determines your happiness.
Committing to these understandings, one will embody a boost in immunity, balanced metabolism, better sleep, a boost in sexual performance, weight reduction, increased energy and vitality.
I am humbled and forever grateful for the opportunities given, and currently offered, to teach the timelessness gift of Yoga.

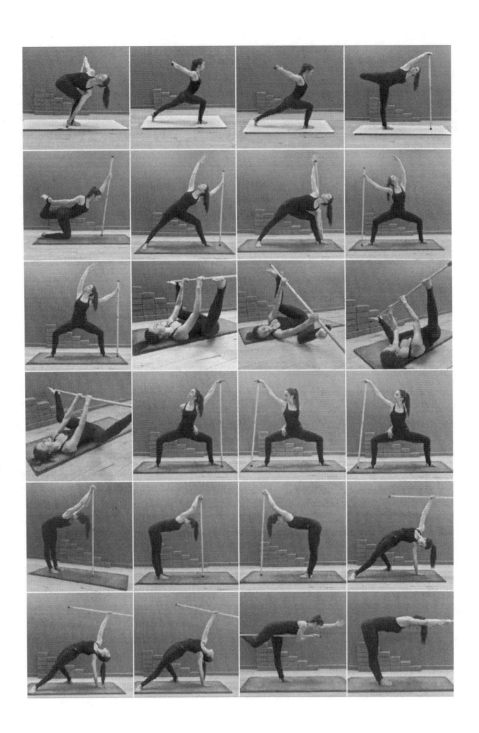

make time for yourself.

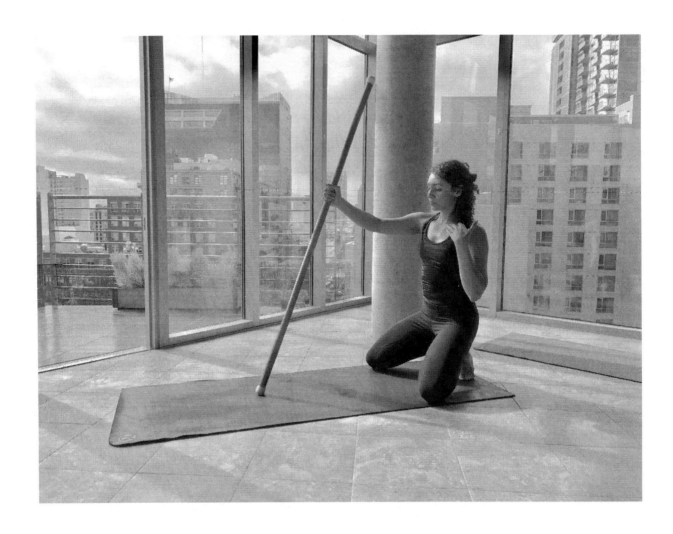

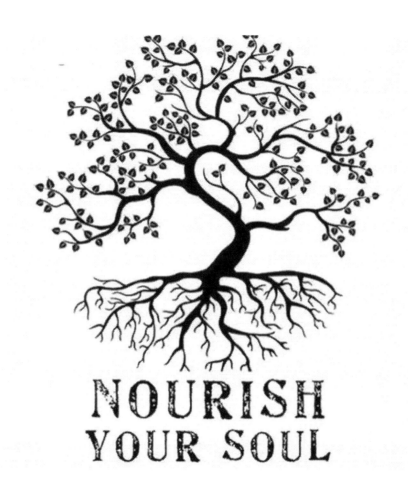

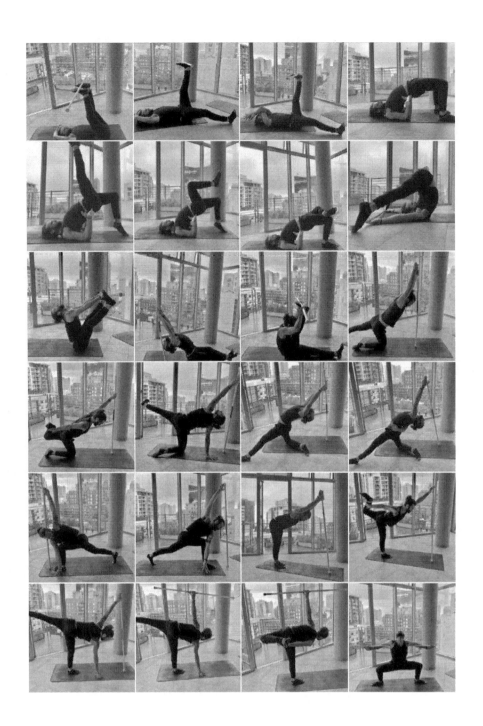

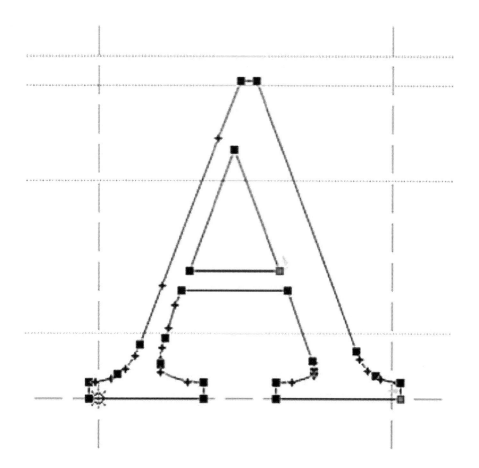

<u>Acceptance</u>

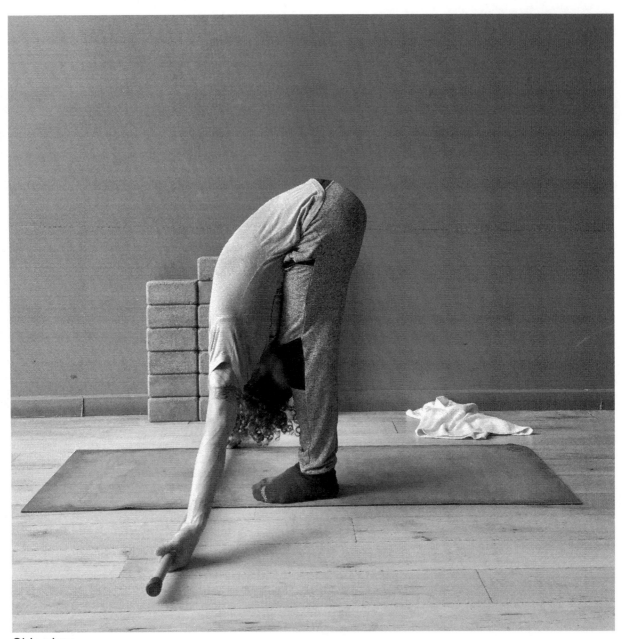
Side view

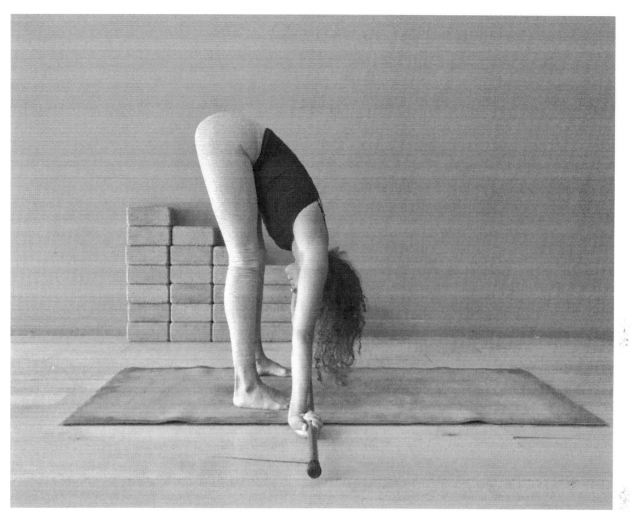
Side view

3

<u>Albatross</u>

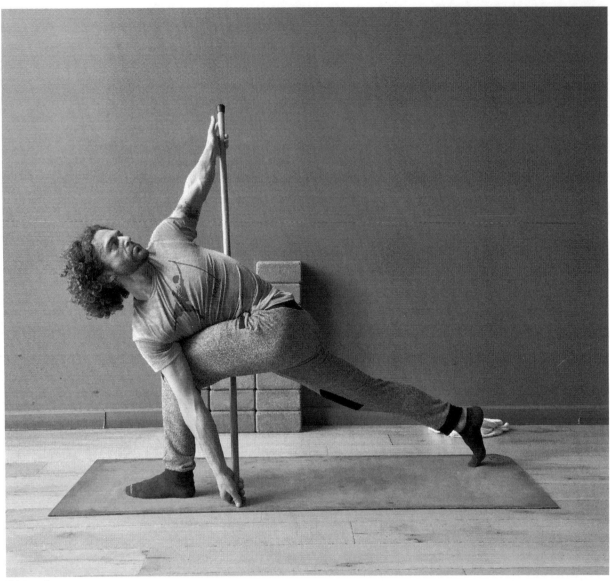

Side view

4

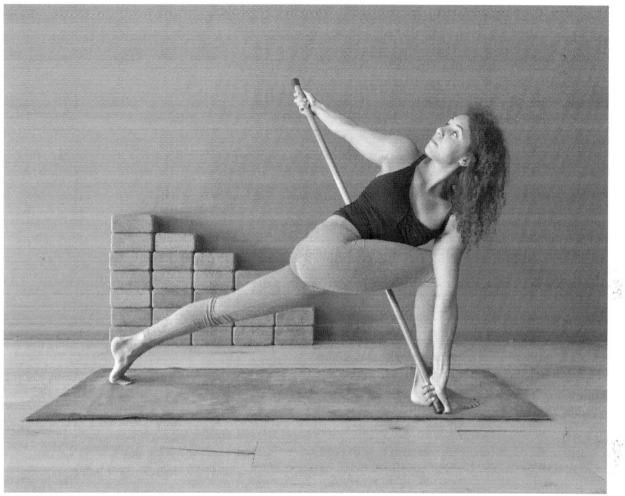
Side view

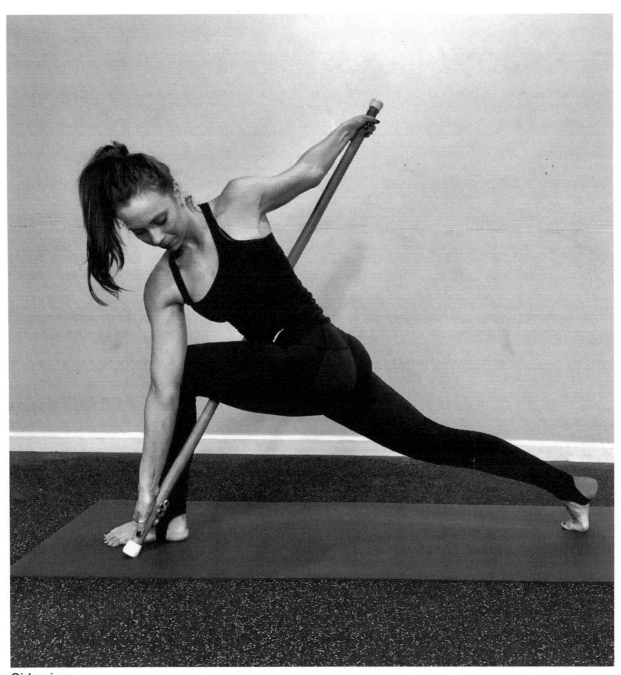
Side view

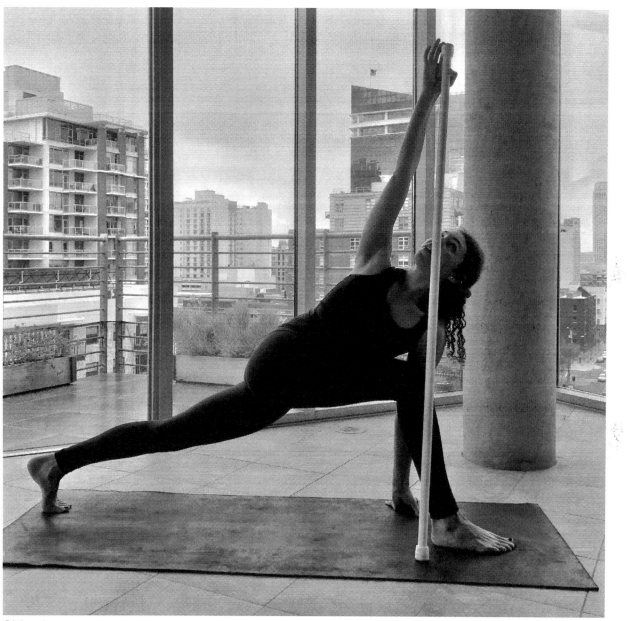
Side view

Angel Fish

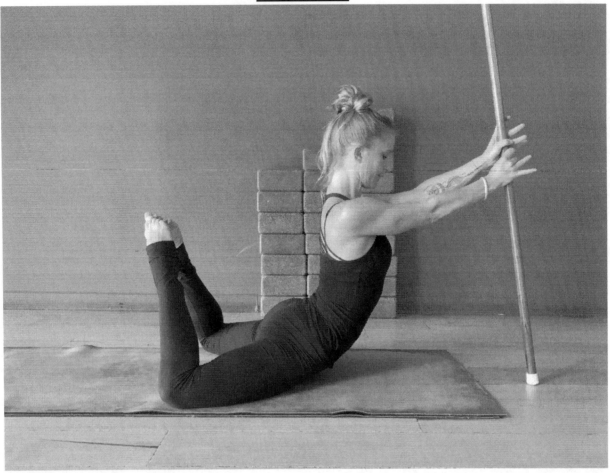

Side view

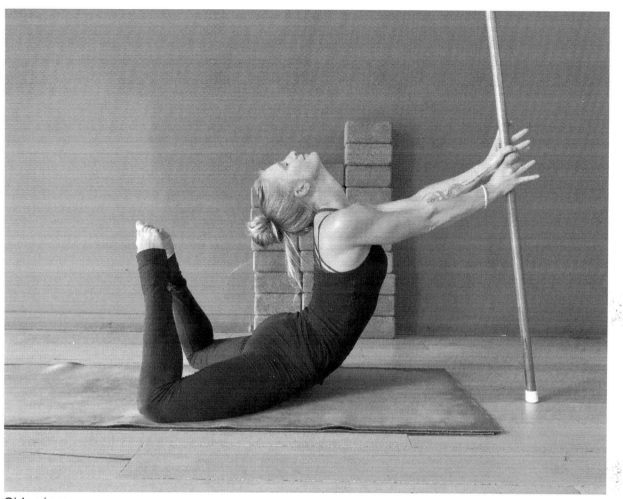

Side view

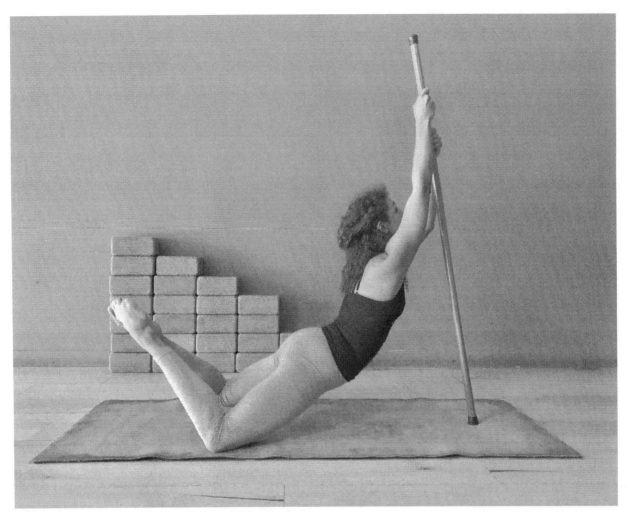
Side view

10

Archer

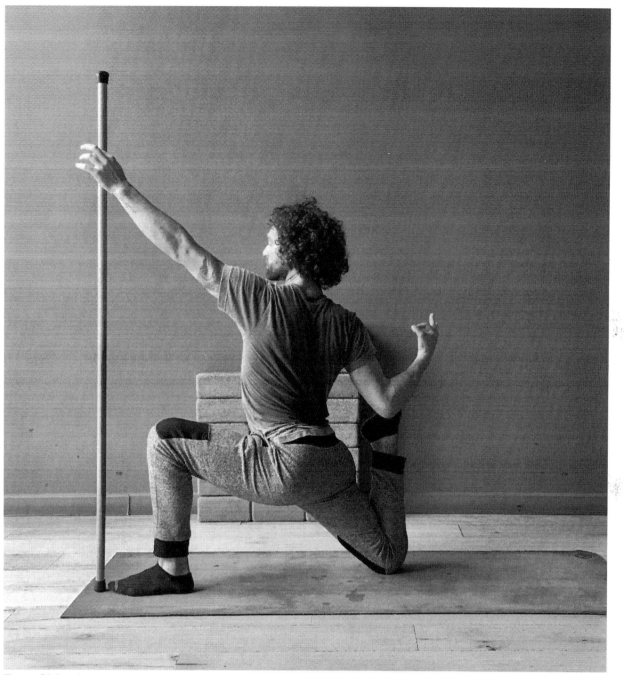

Rear Side view

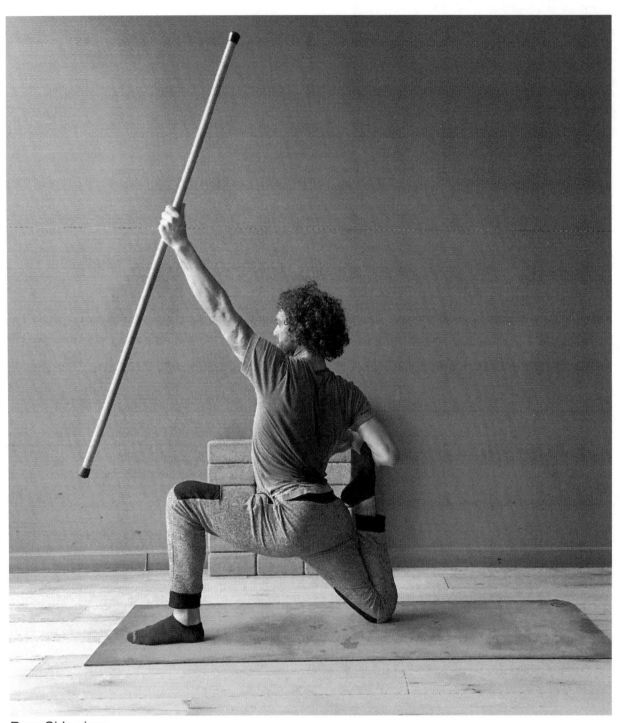

Rear Side view

Arm up the wall

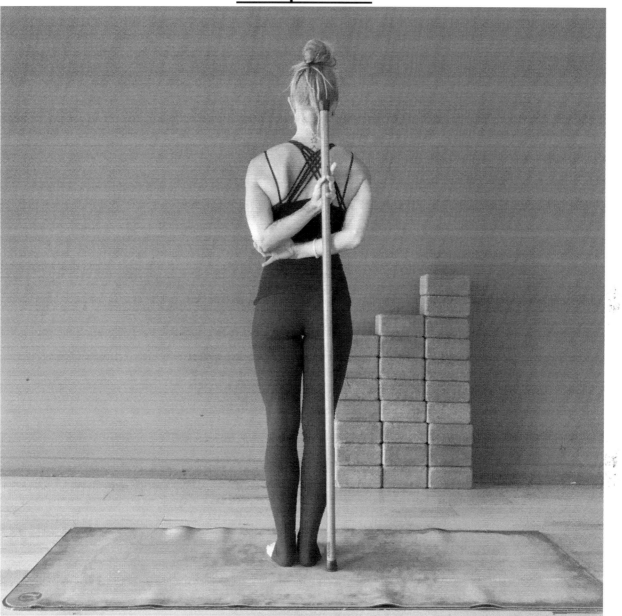

Rear view

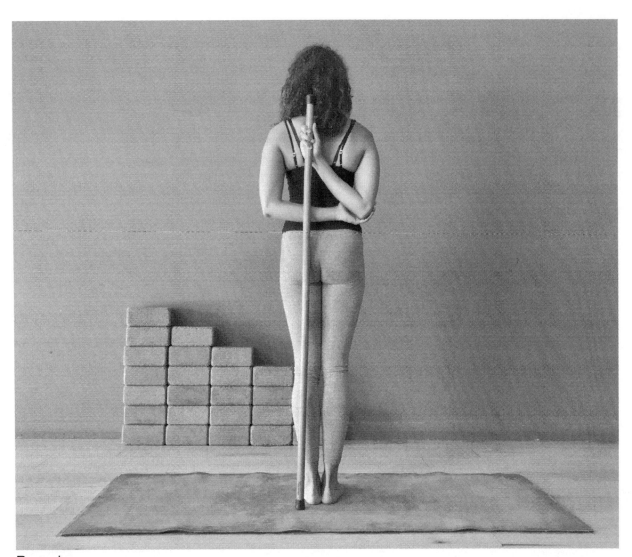
Rear view

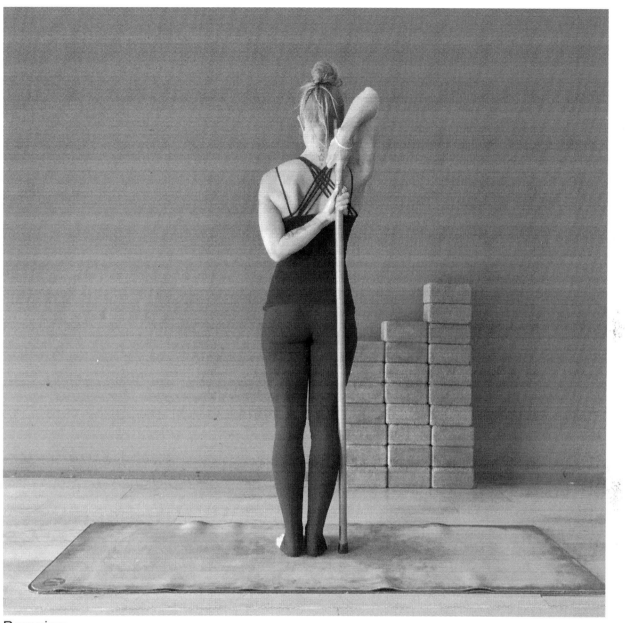

Rear view

Asian Elephant

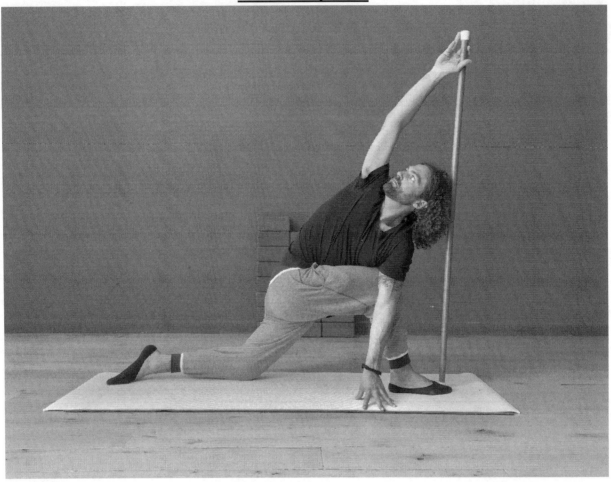

Side view

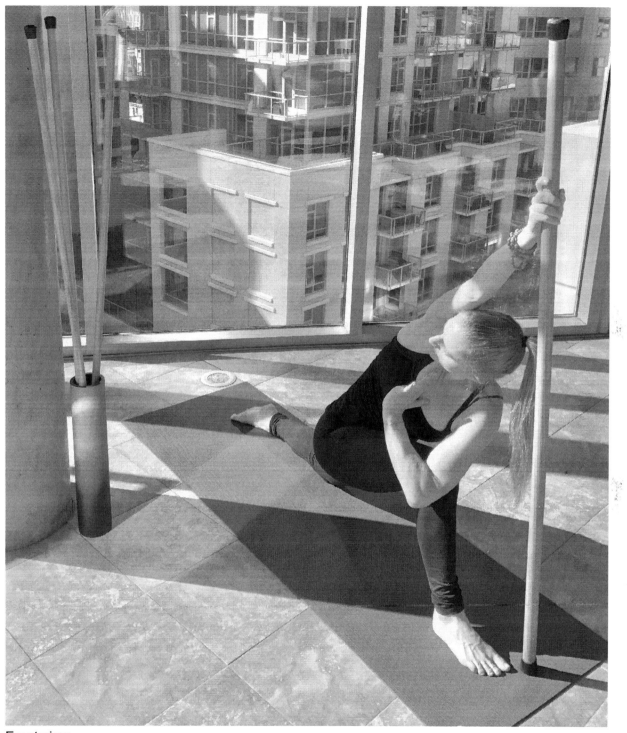

Front view

Aurora

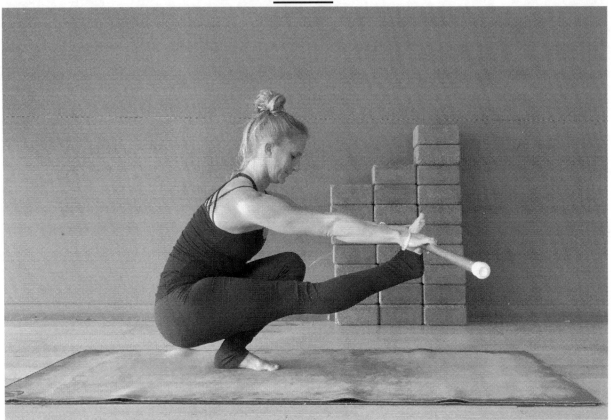

Side view

Axis

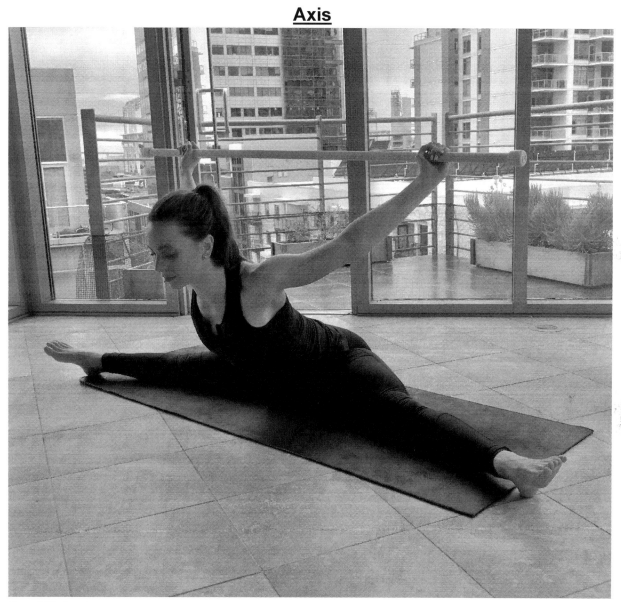

Front Side view

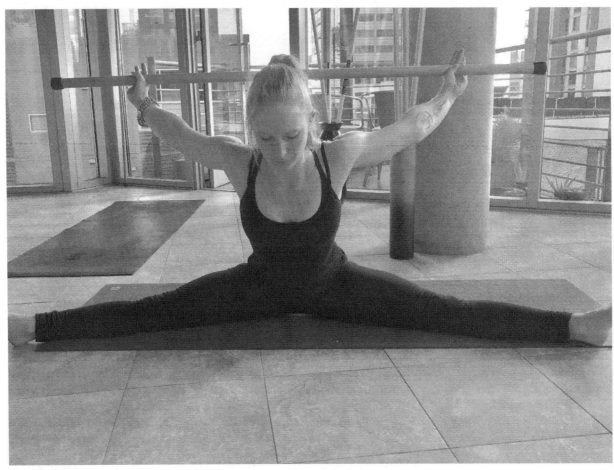

Front view

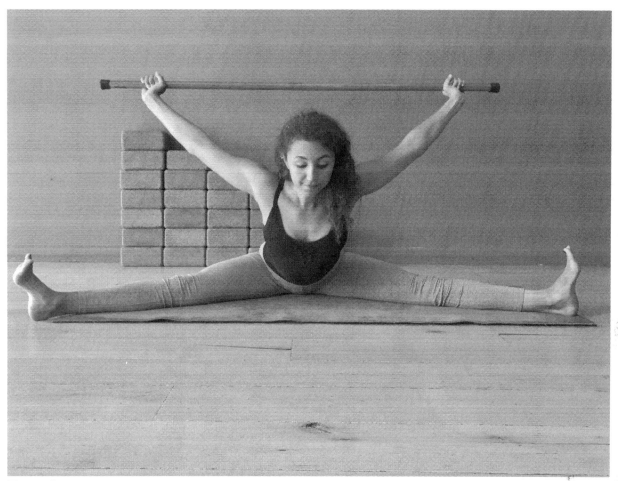

Front view

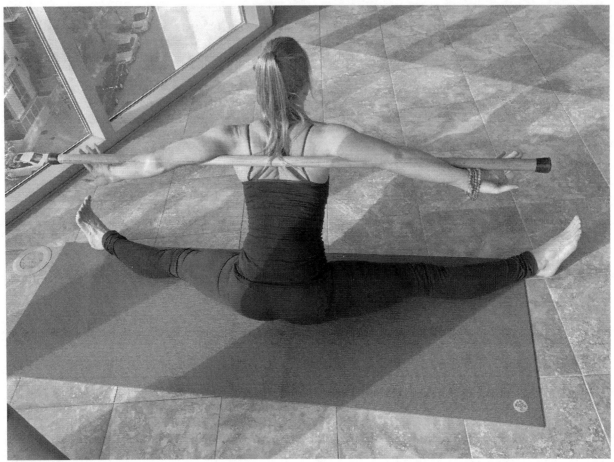
Rear view

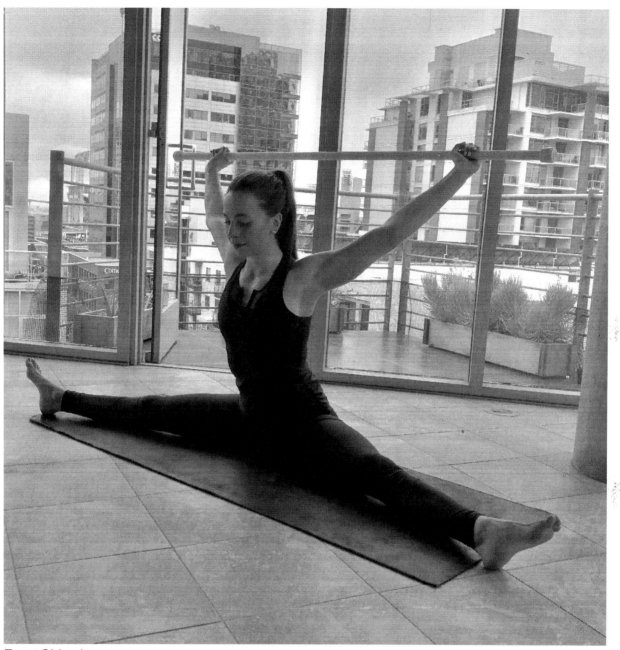
Front Side view

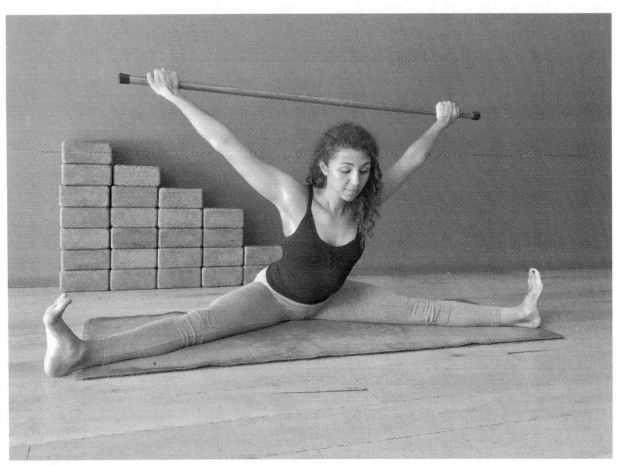
Front Side view

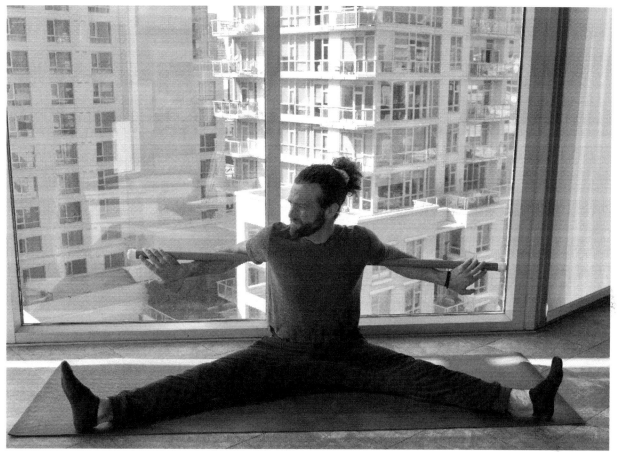

Front view

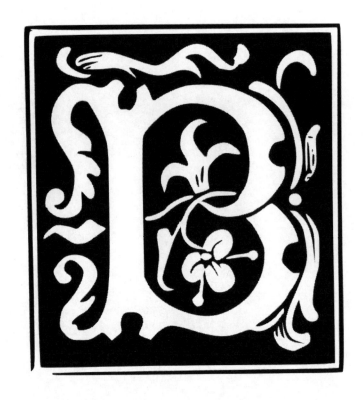

Baby Crow

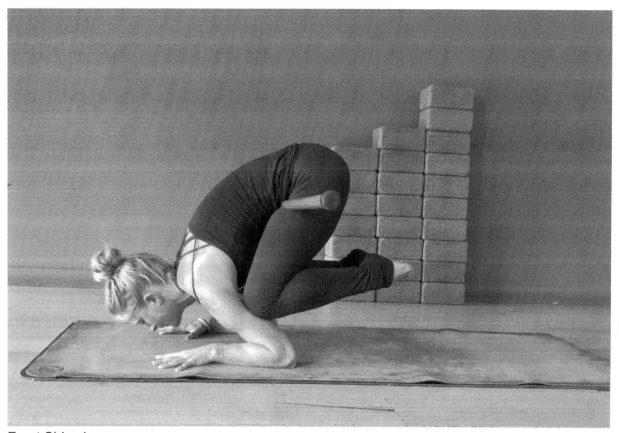
Front Side view

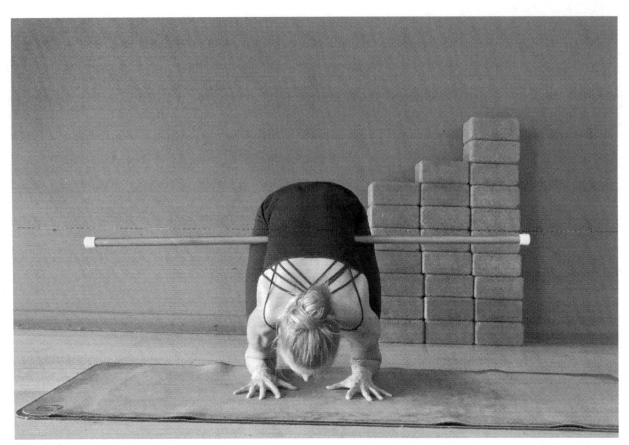
Front view

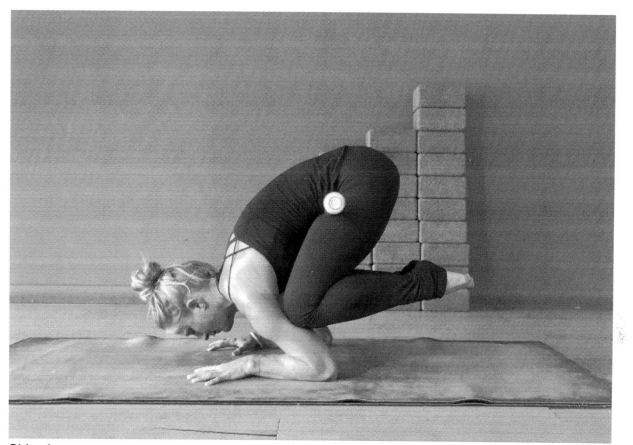

Side view

29

<u>Ballerina</u>

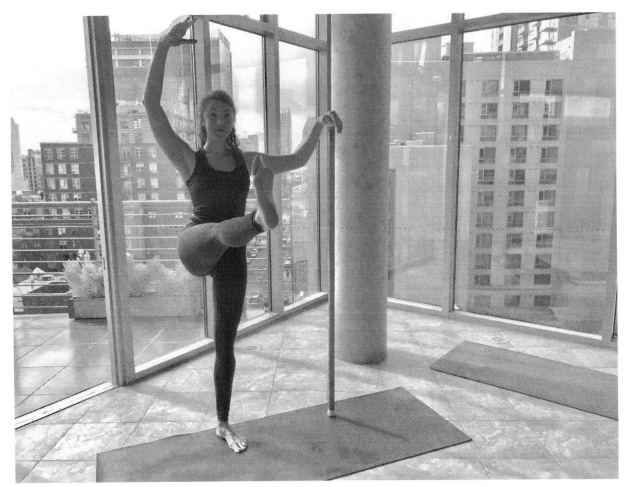

Front view

Barracuda

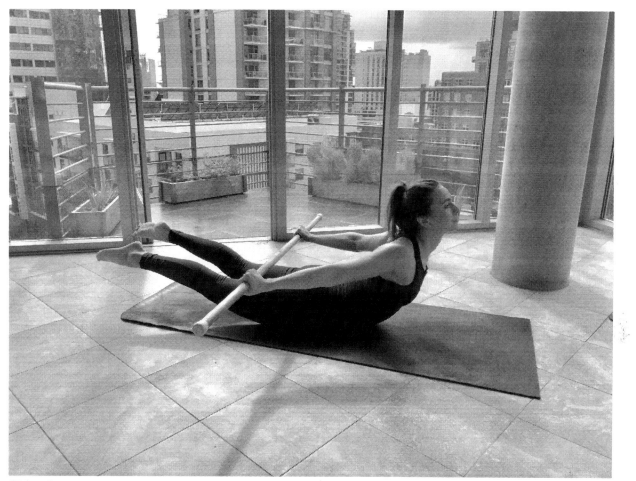

Side view

Bind and Balance

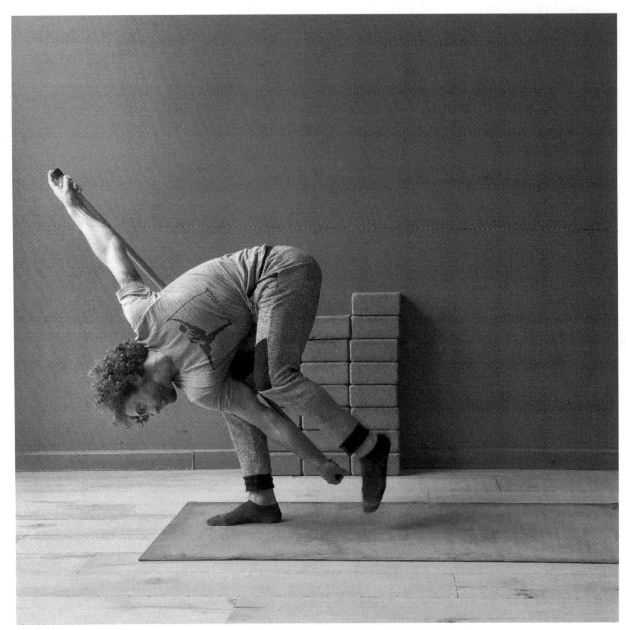
Side view

Birds of Paradise

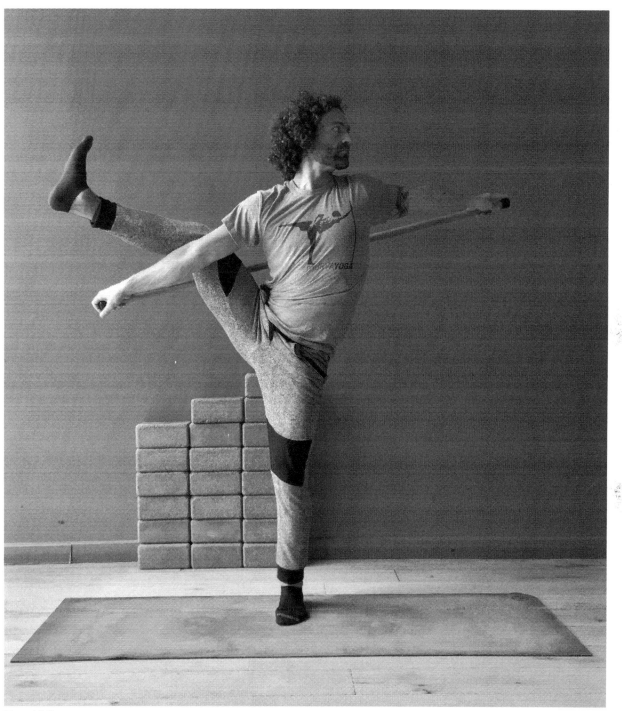

Front View

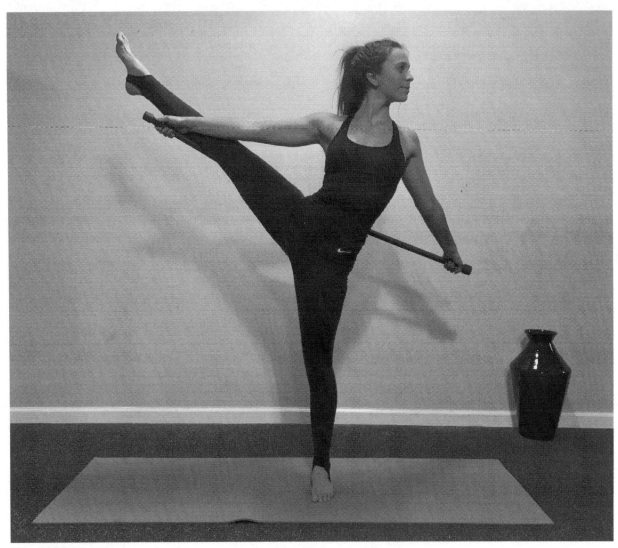

Front View

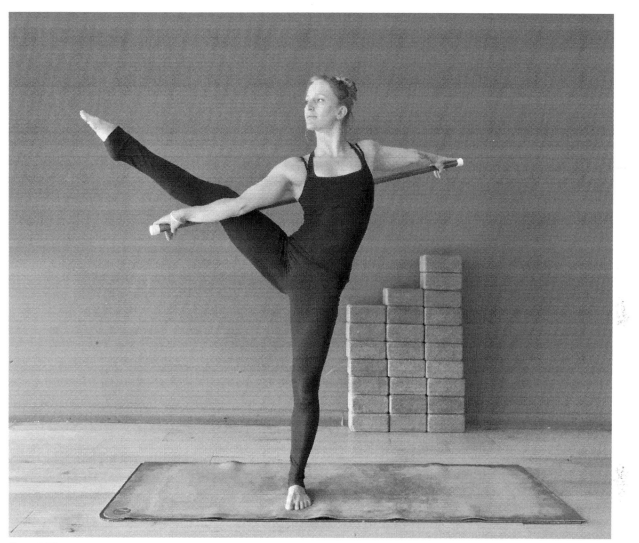
Front View

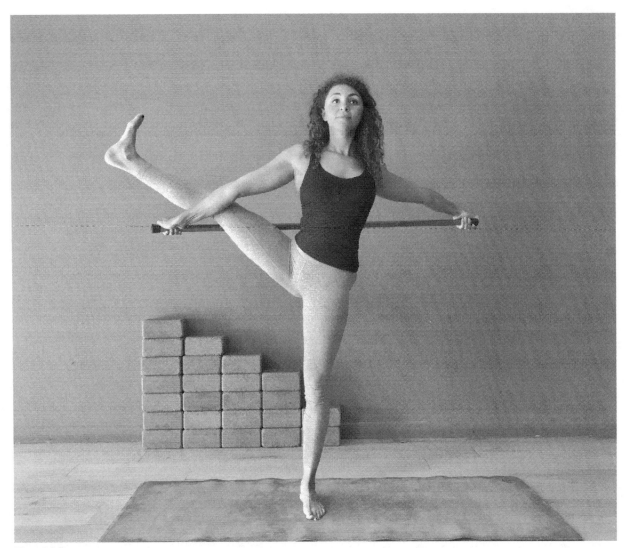

Front View

Black Moon

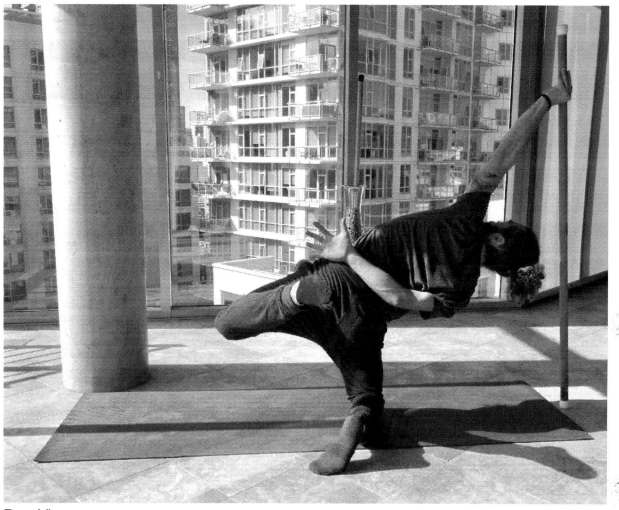

Rear View

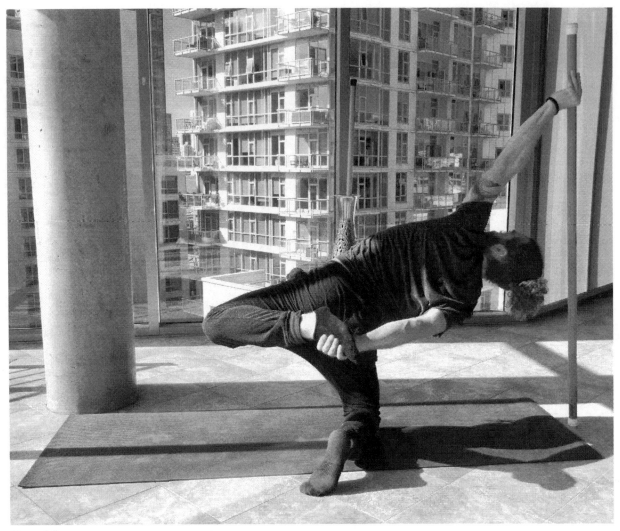

Rear View

Bliss on Tap

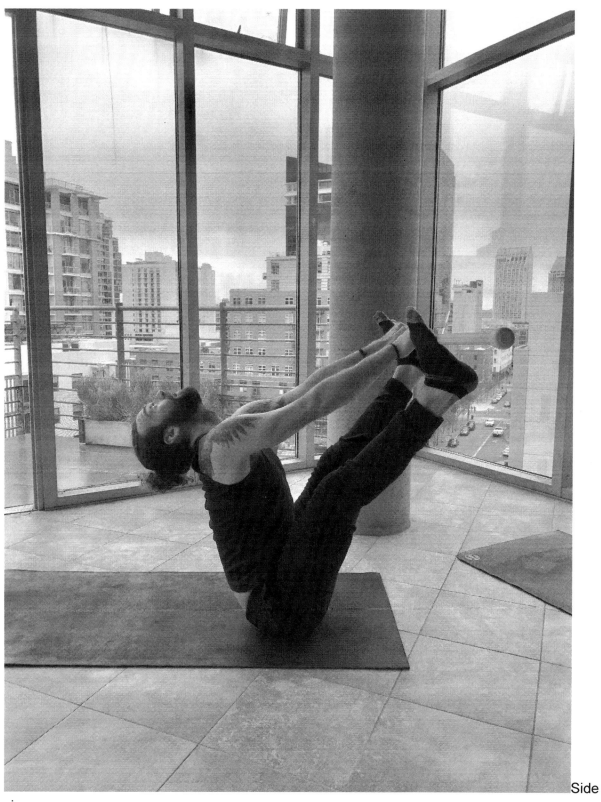

Side view

Bloom & Prosper

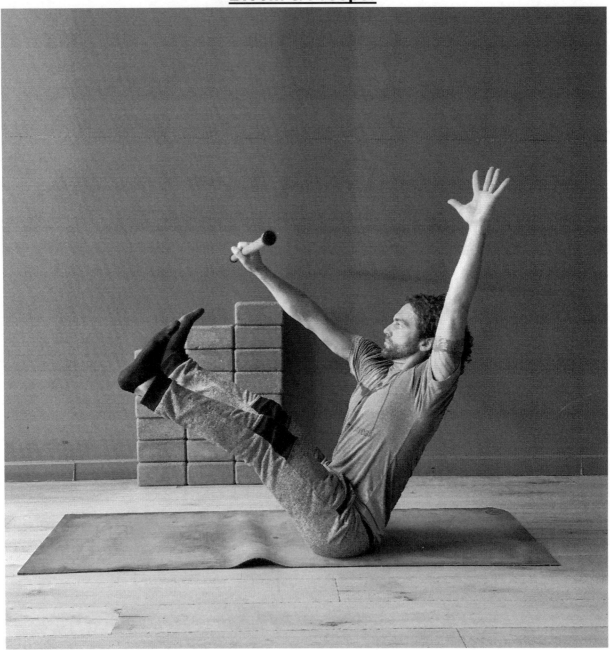

Side view

Boat

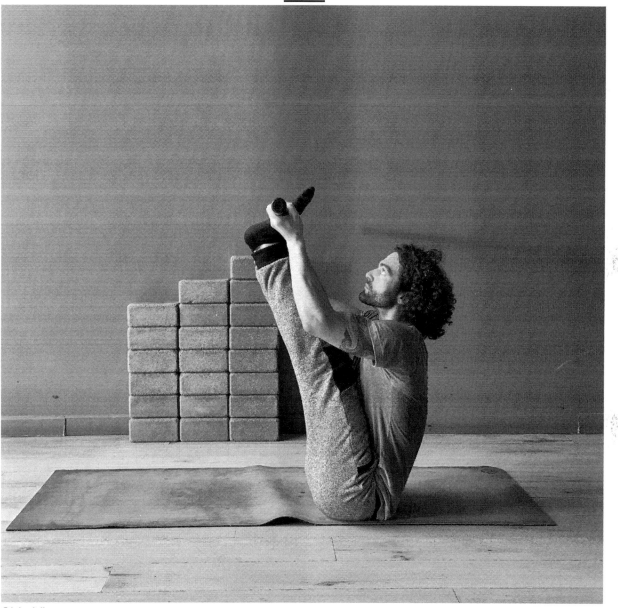

Side View

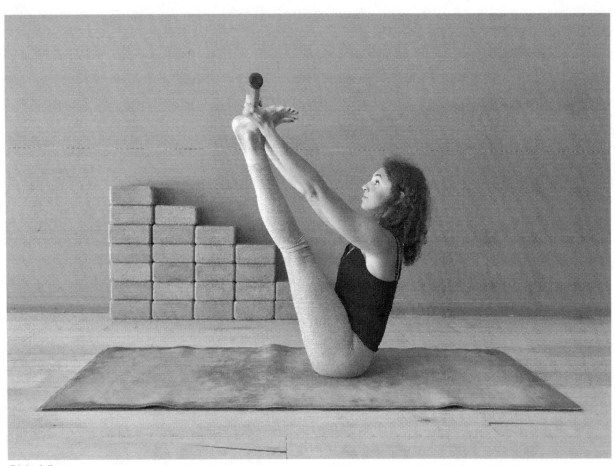

Side View

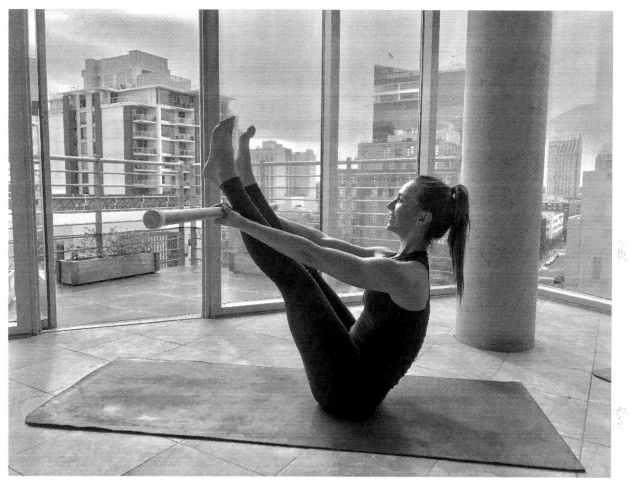

Side view

43

<u>Bridge</u>

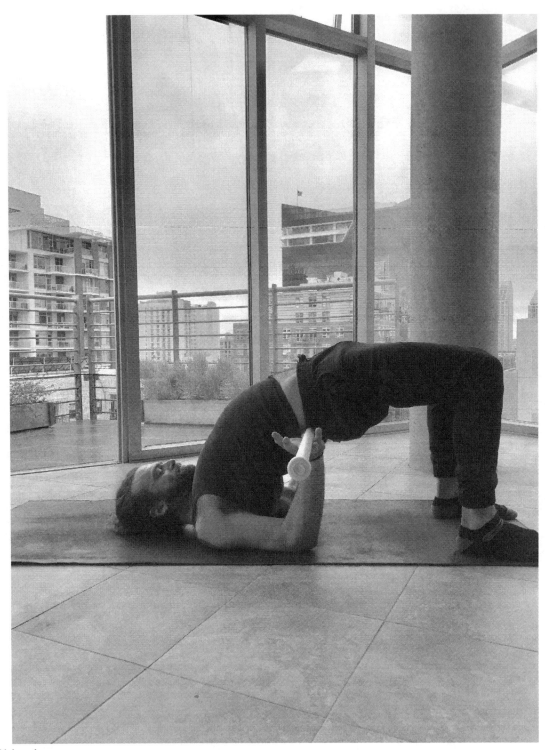

Side view

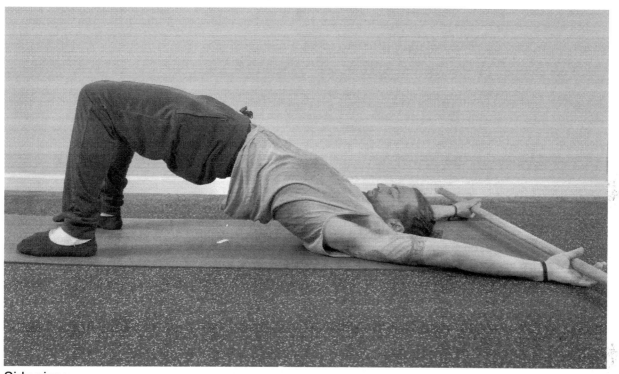

Side view

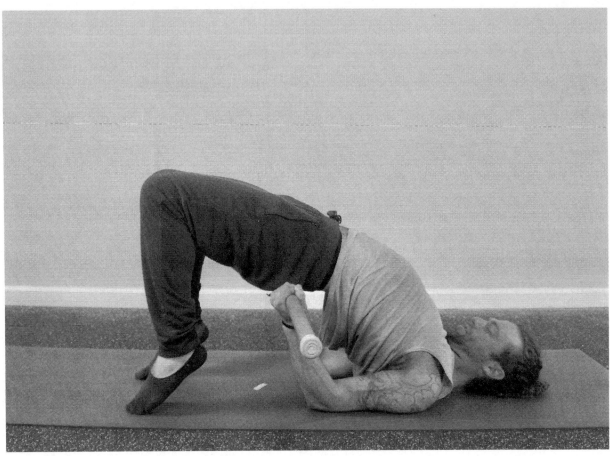
Side view

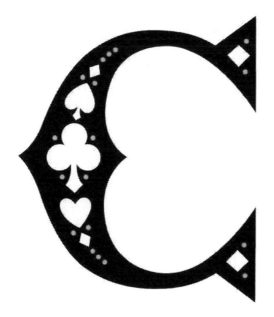

Camel

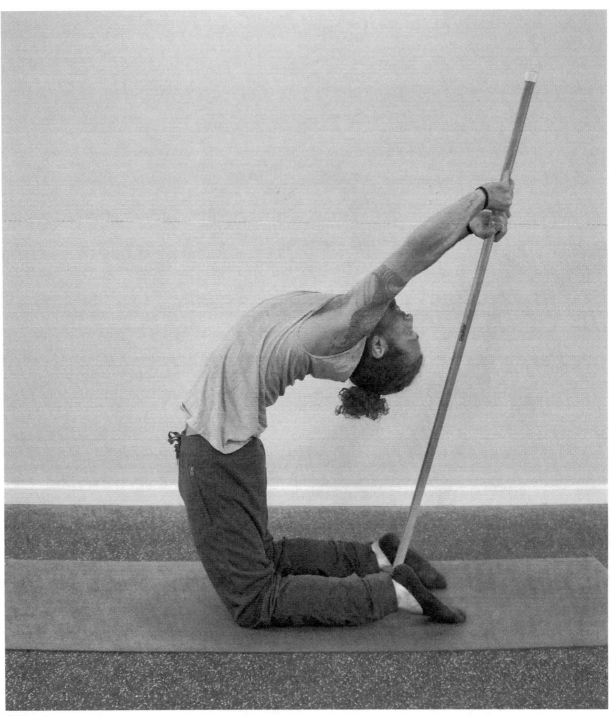

Side view

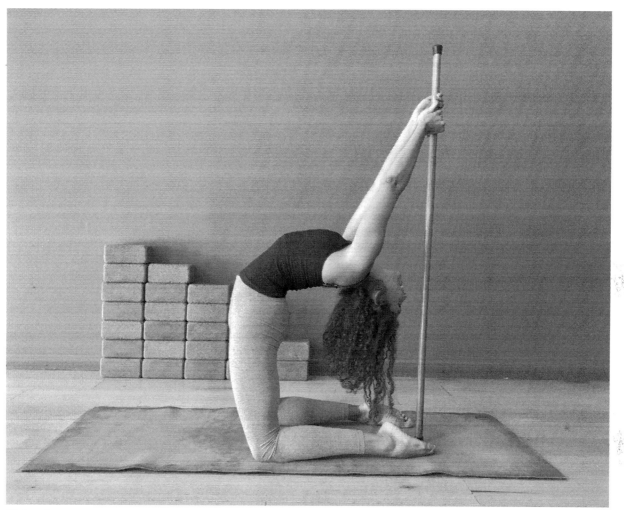

Side view

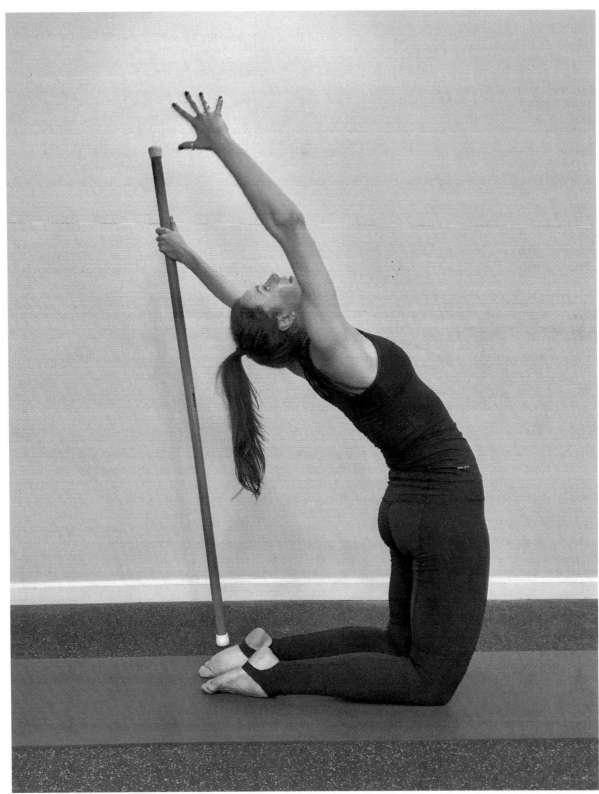
Side view

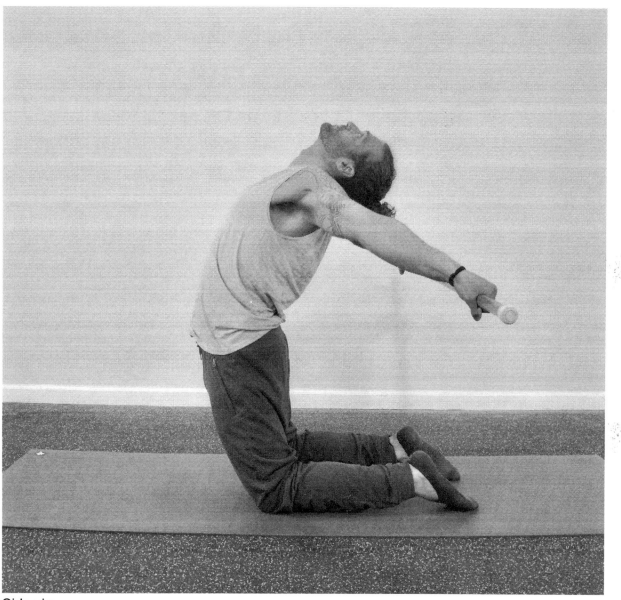
Side view

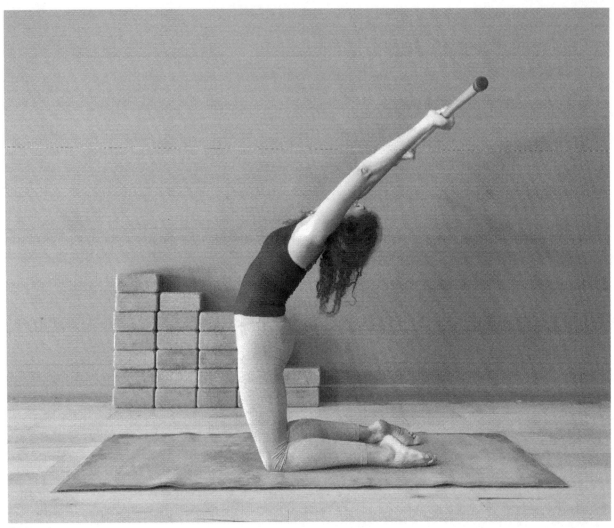

Side view

52

Capricorn

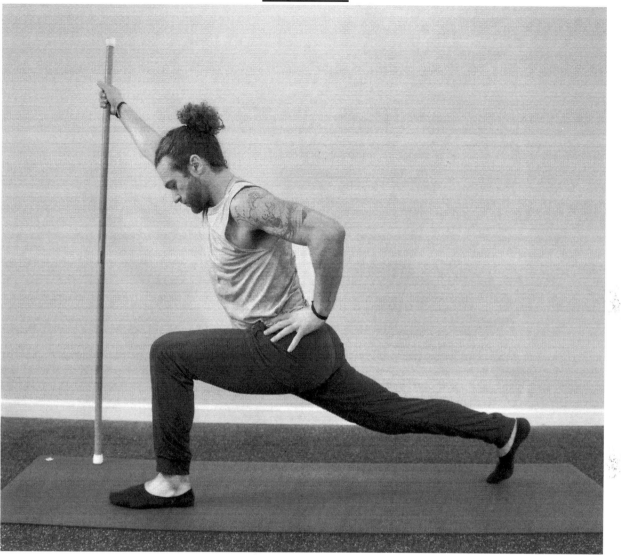

Side view

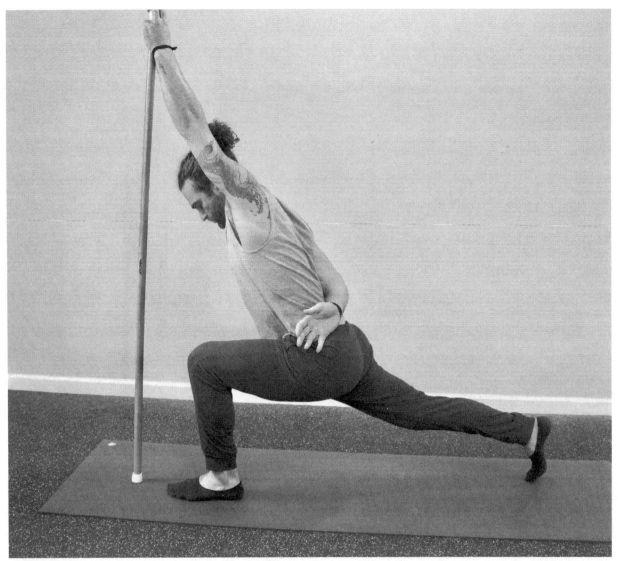
Side view

Chair

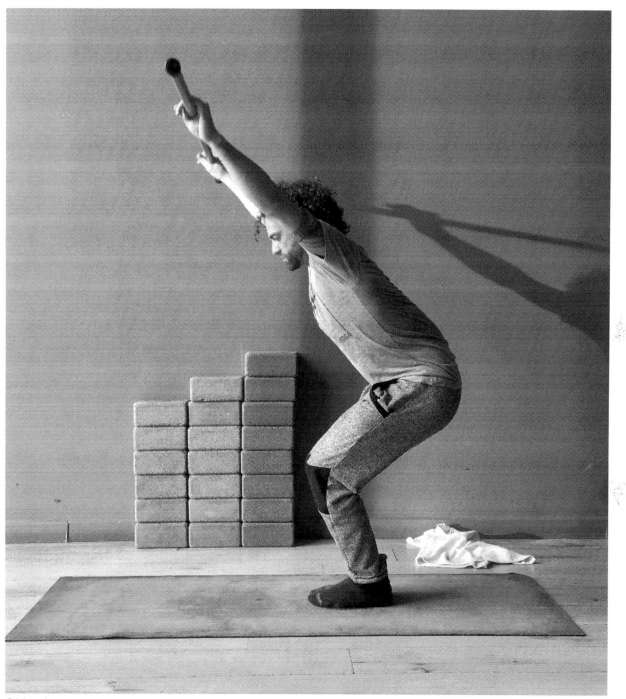

Side view

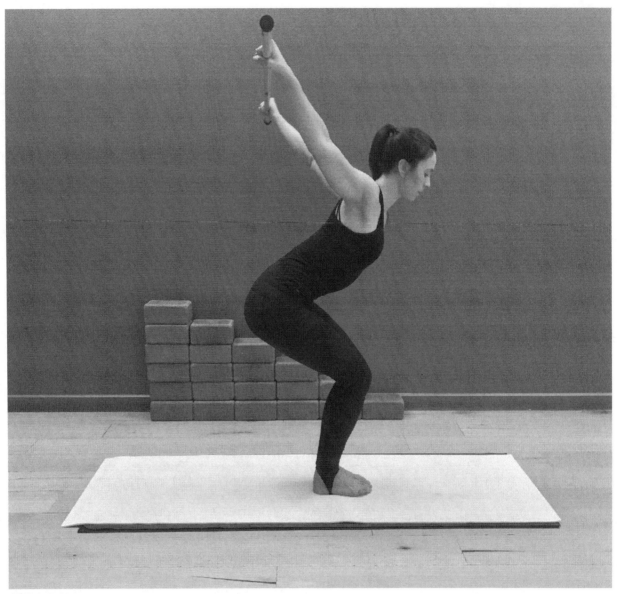

Side view

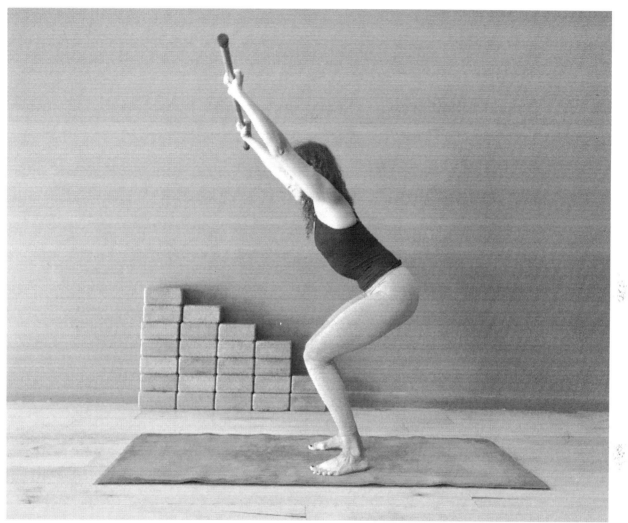
Side view

Challenging

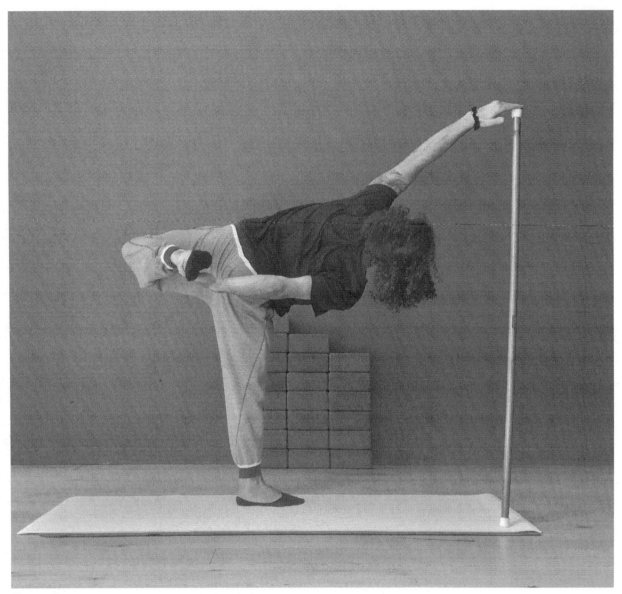

Rear view

58

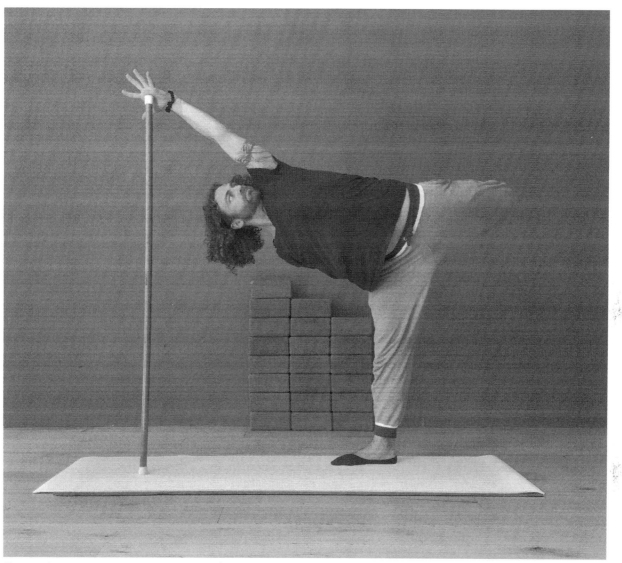

Front view

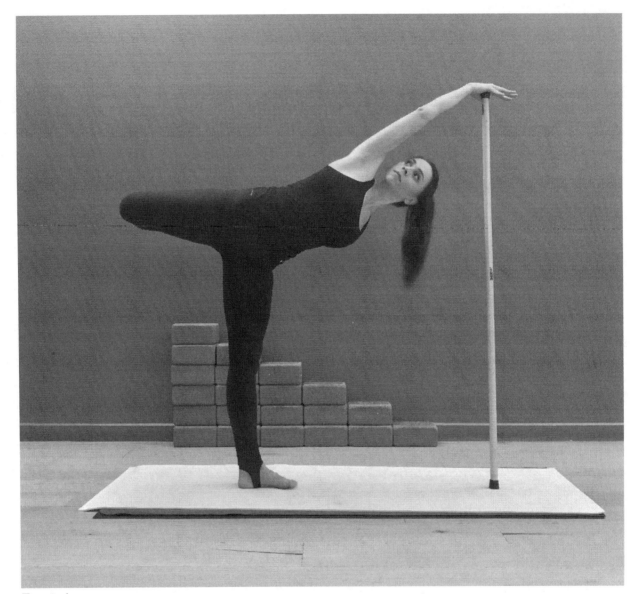
Front view

60

Champion

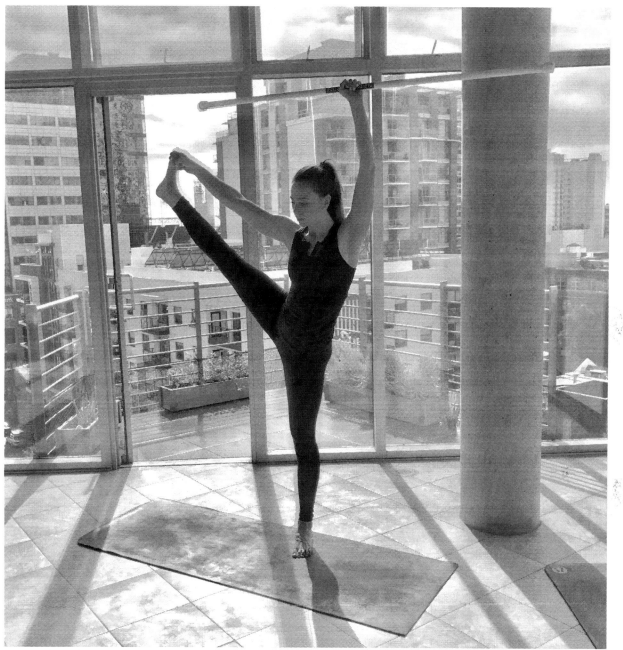
Front side view

Child's Pose

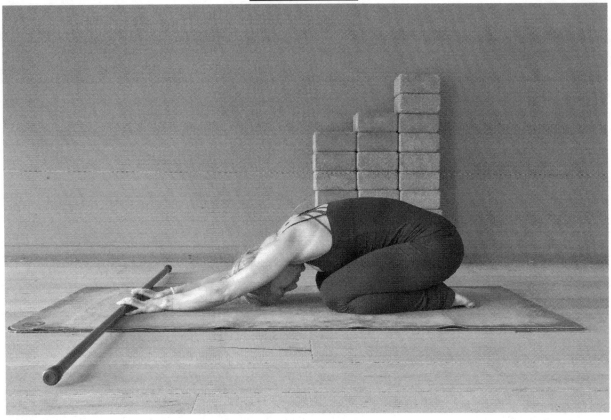

Side view

Comet

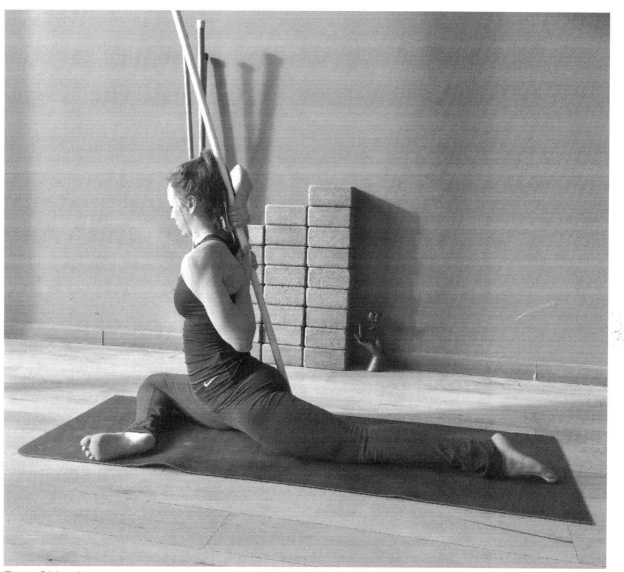

Rear Side view

Crescent

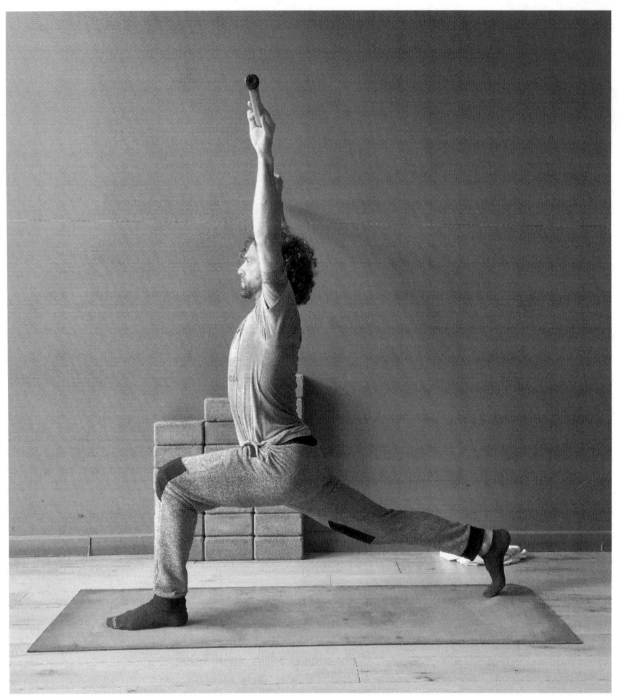

Side view

64

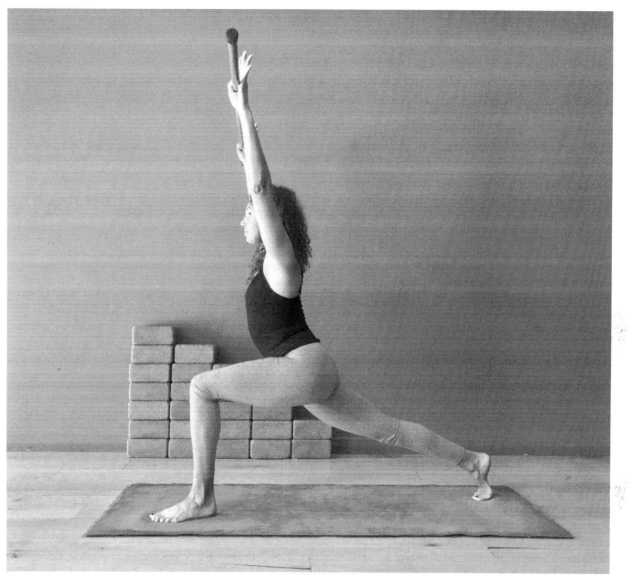
Side view

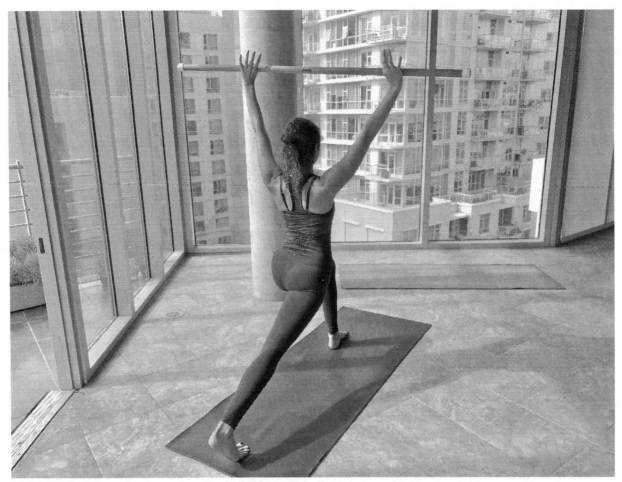

Rear Side view

Crow

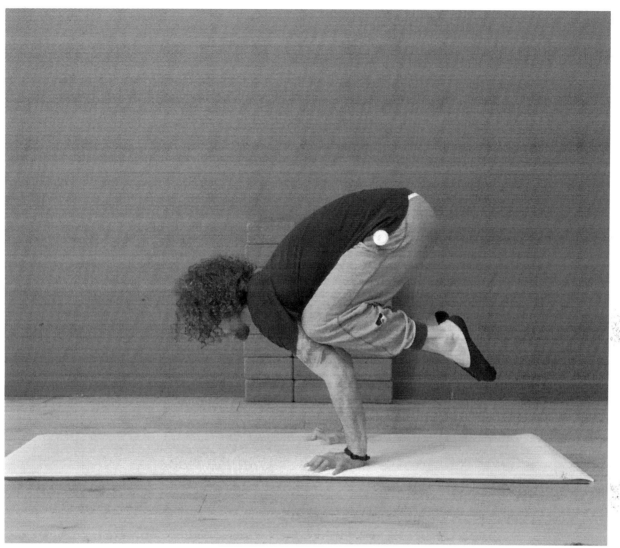

Side view

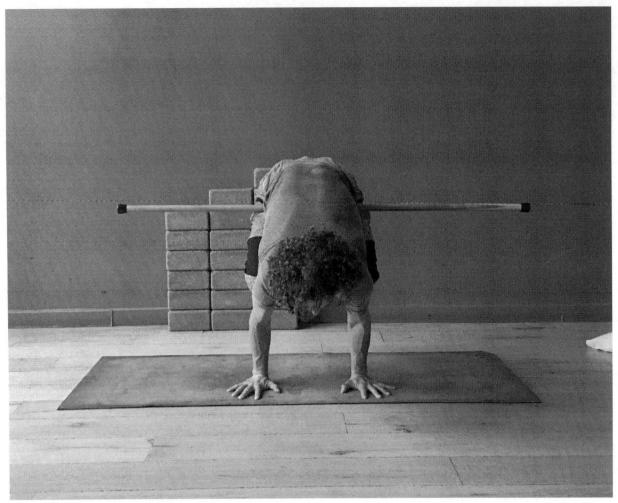

Front view

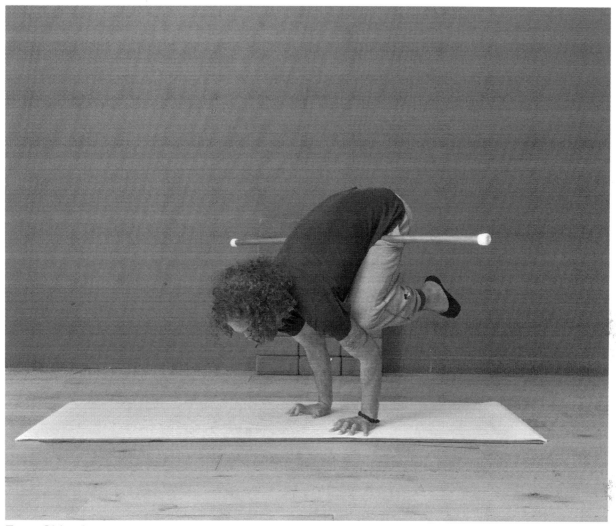

Front Side view

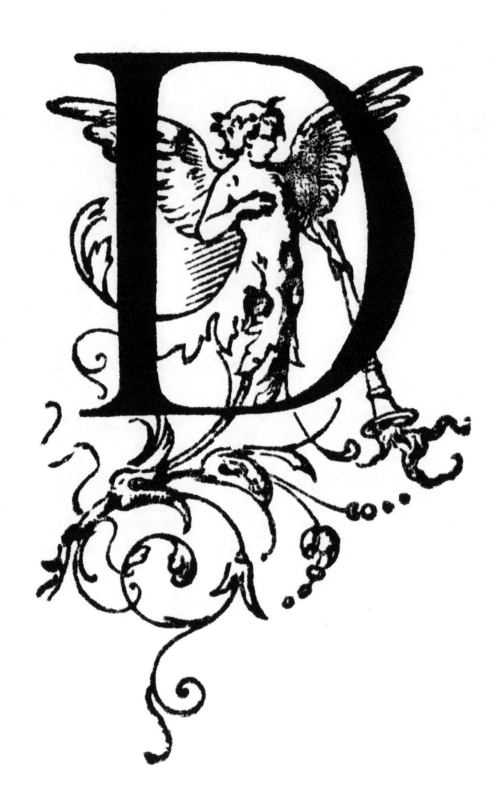

Dancers

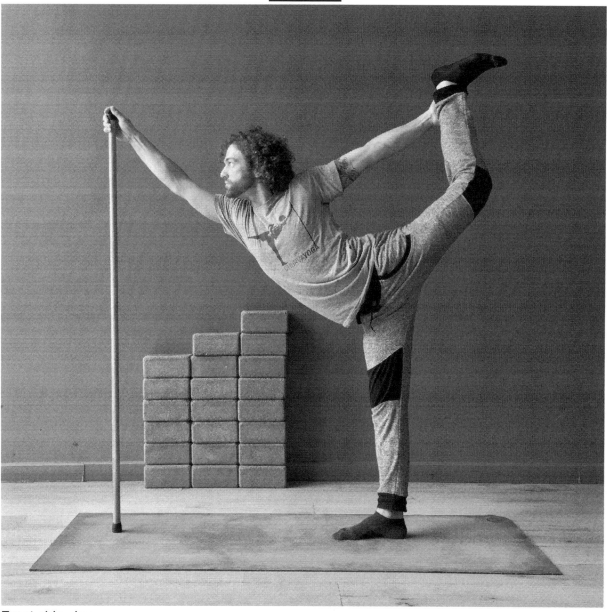

Front side view

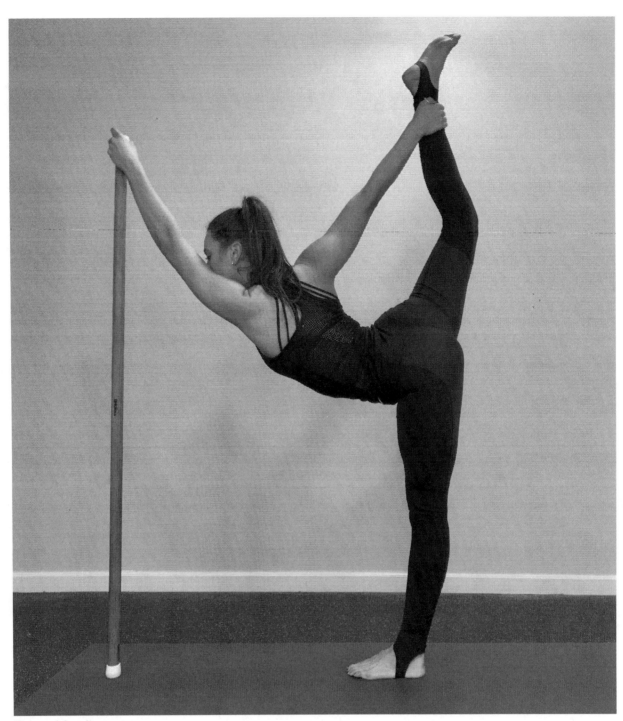

Rear side view

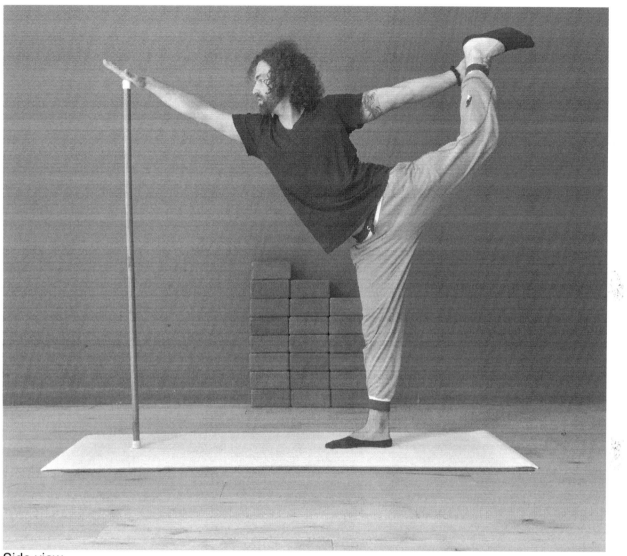

Side view

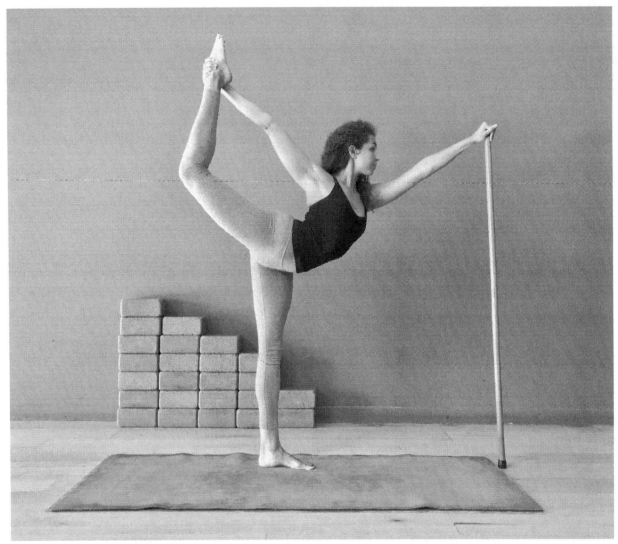
Side view

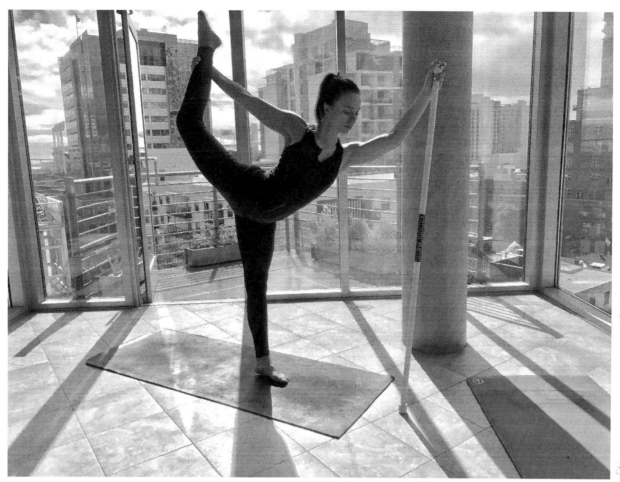

Front side view

Daring

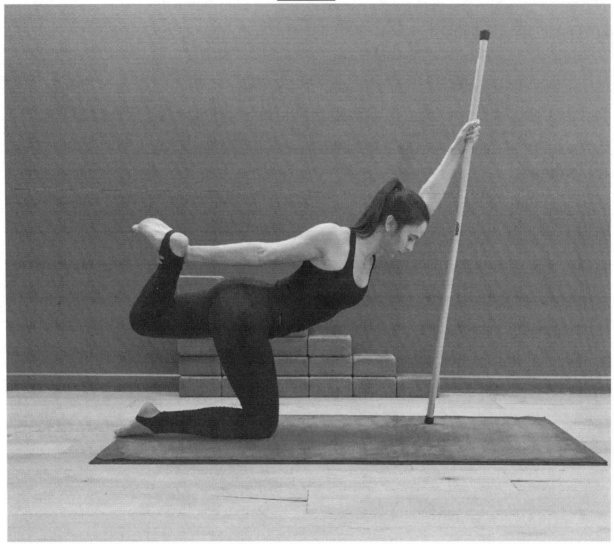

Side view

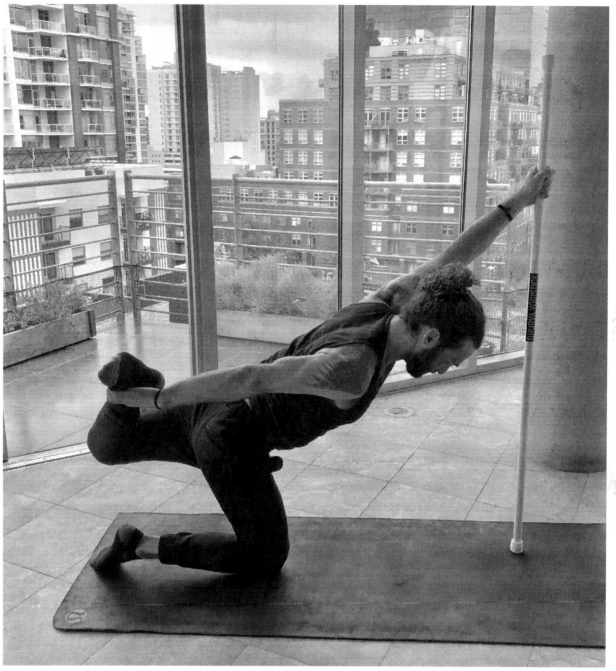

Side view

Deep Pockets

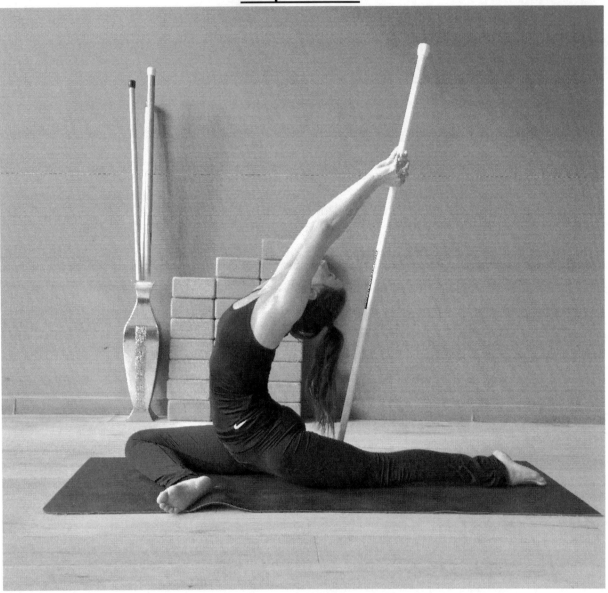

Side view

DeJa Vu

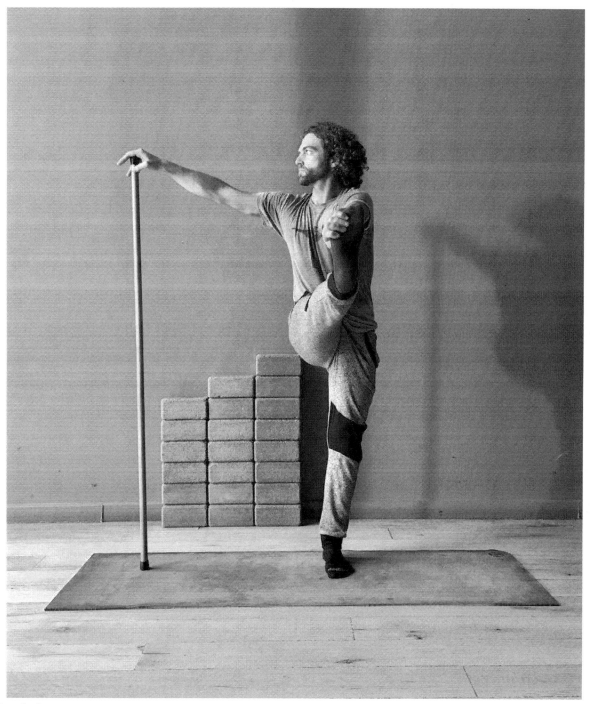

Front view

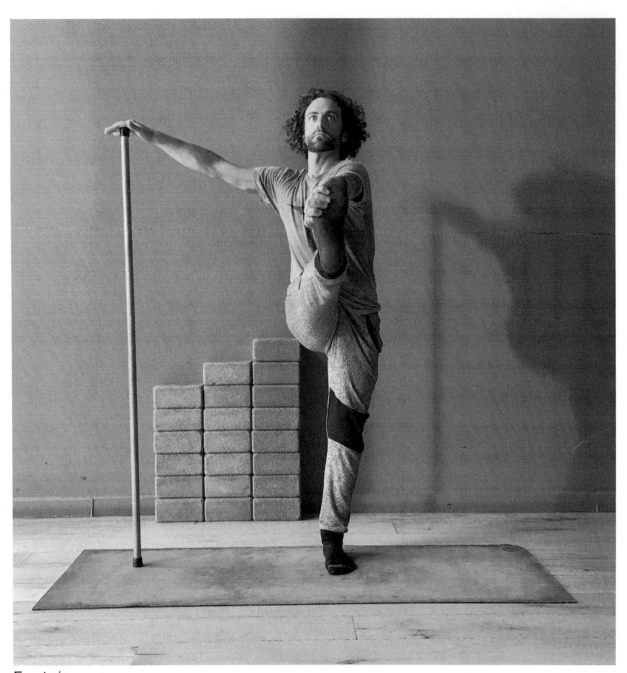
Front view

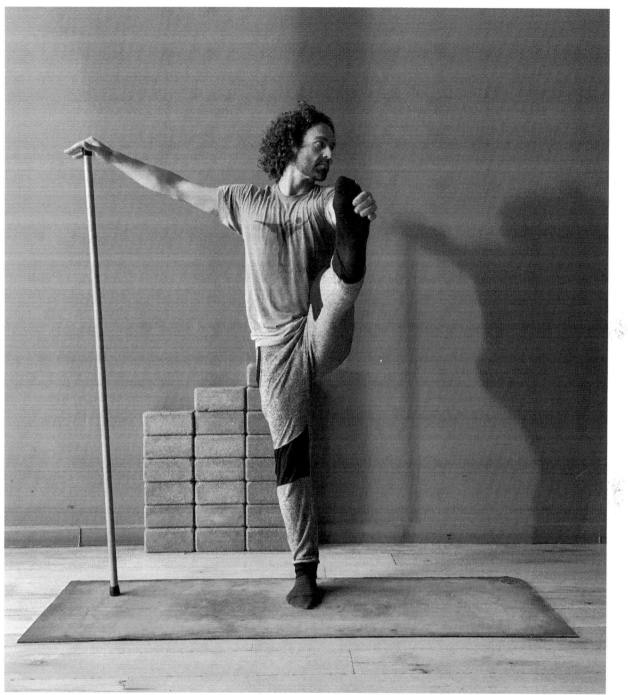

Front view

Dhurva

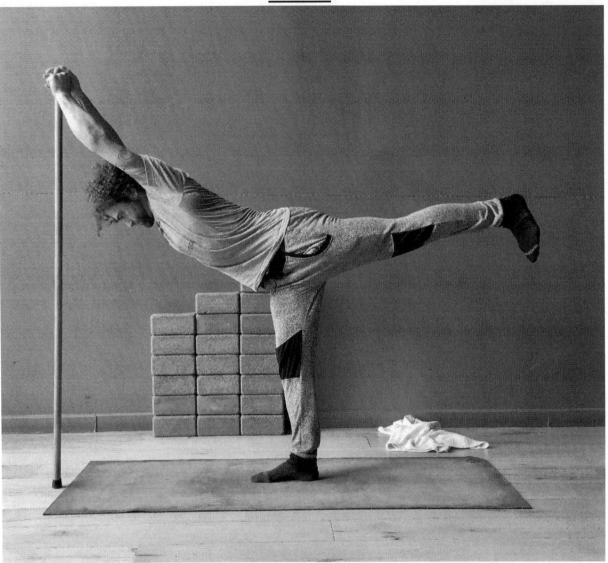

Side view

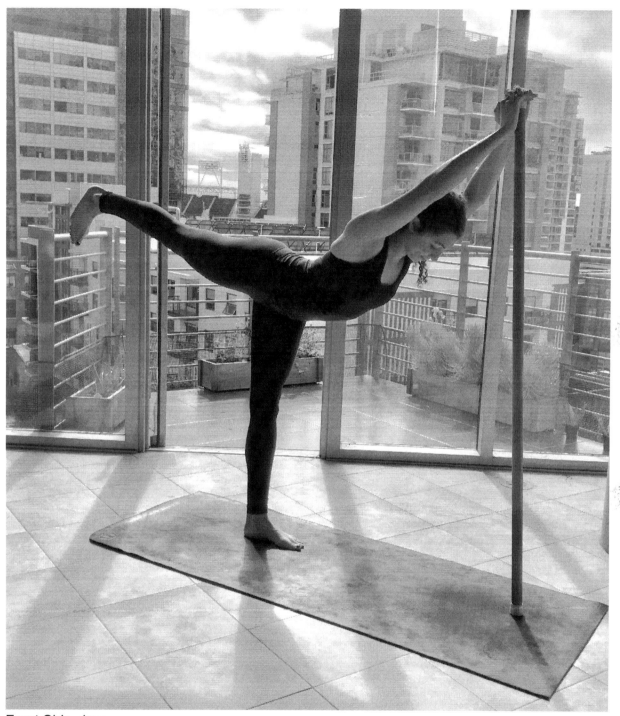

Front Side view

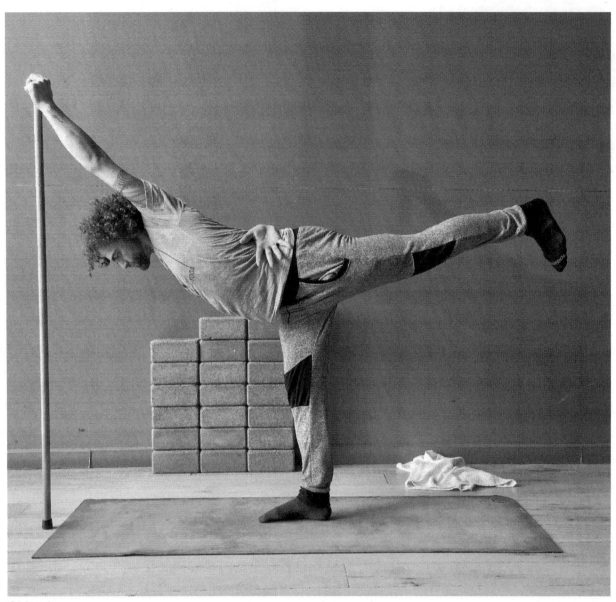
Side view

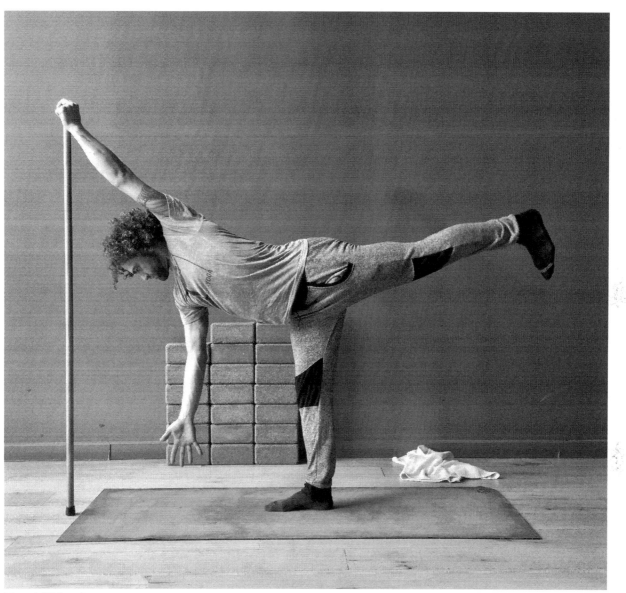

Front Side view

Dhurva Lama

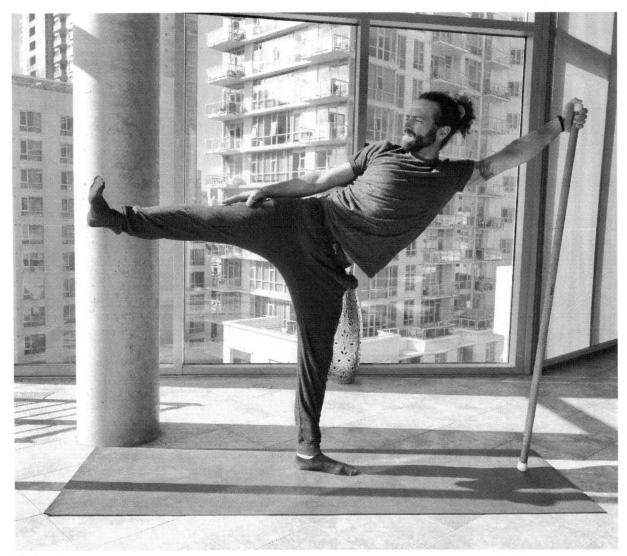

Front view

Double Comet

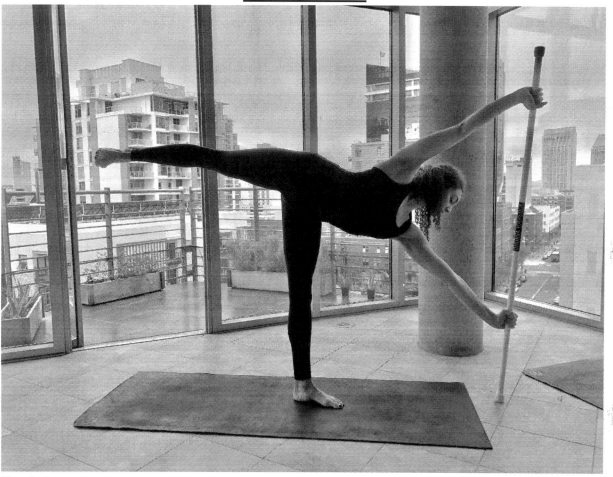

Front view

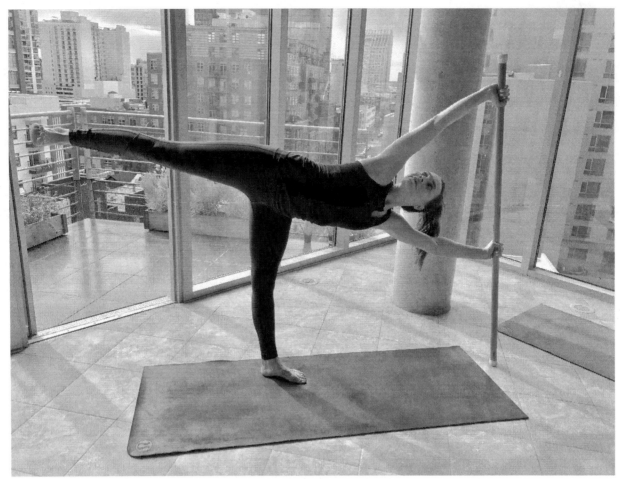

Front view

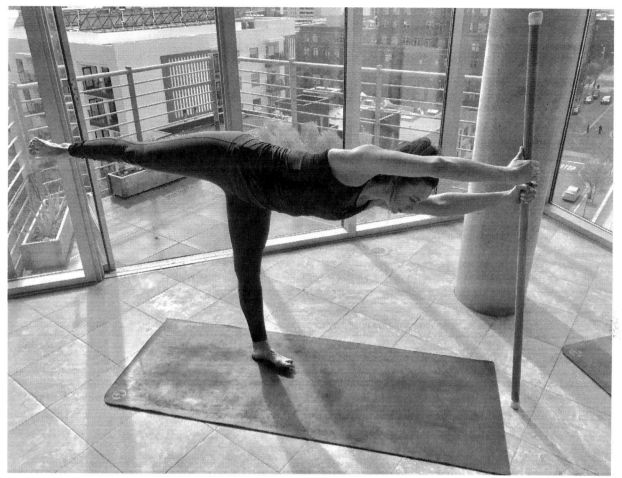

Front Side view

Dreamer

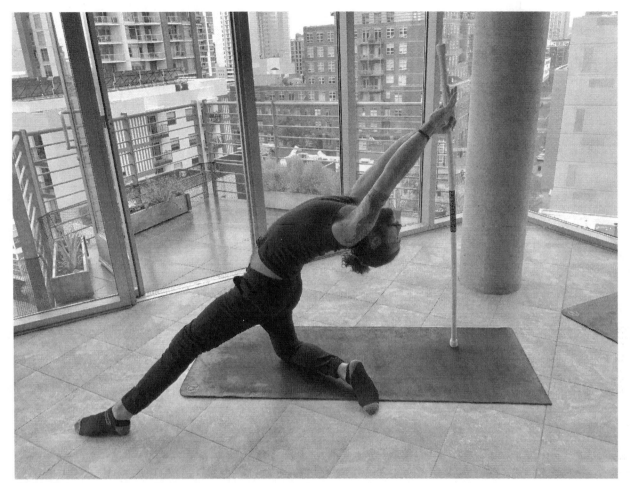
Side view

Duck

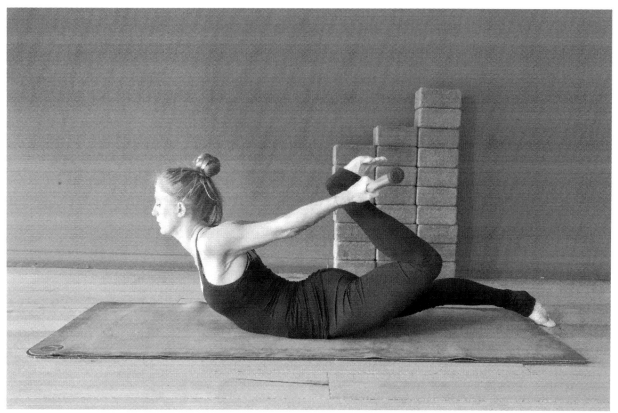

Side view

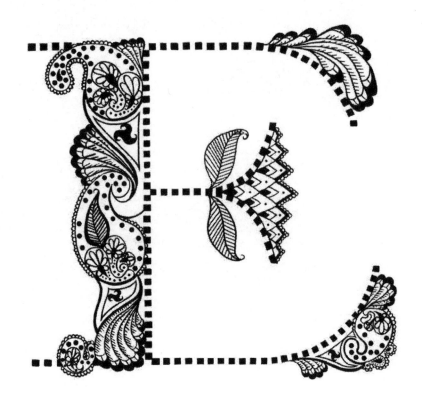

Eagle

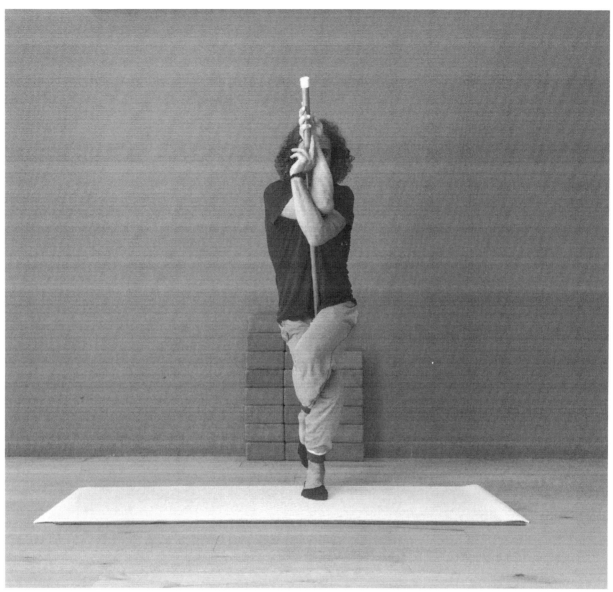

Front view

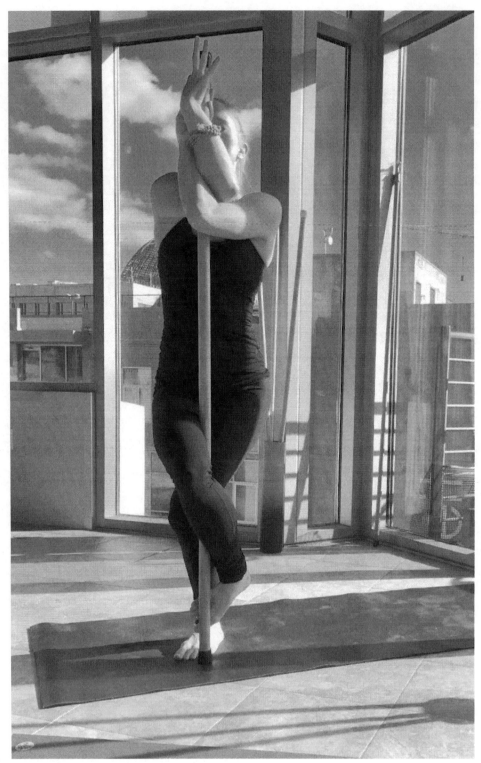

Front view

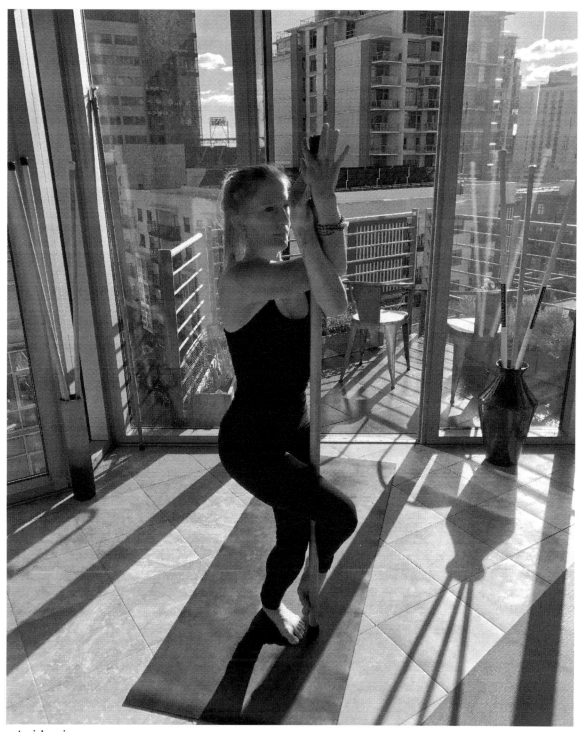
Front side view

Earth

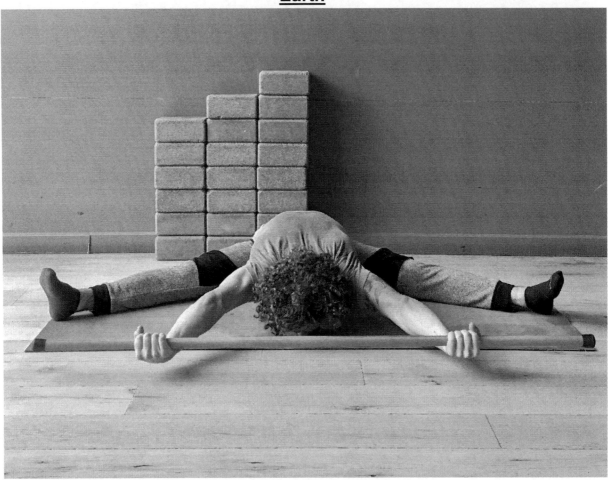

Front view

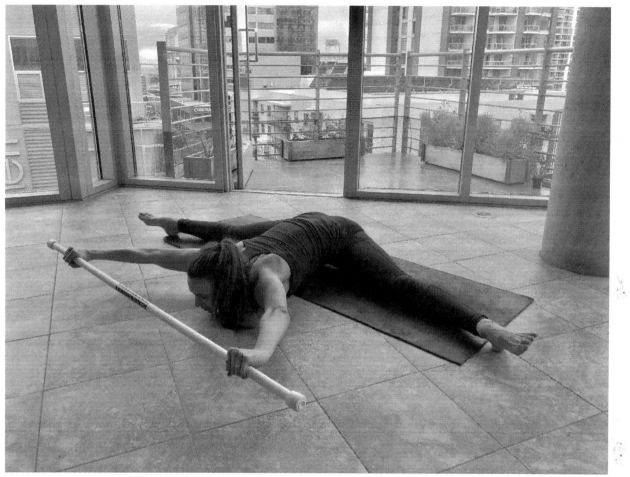
Front Side view

97

Eclipse

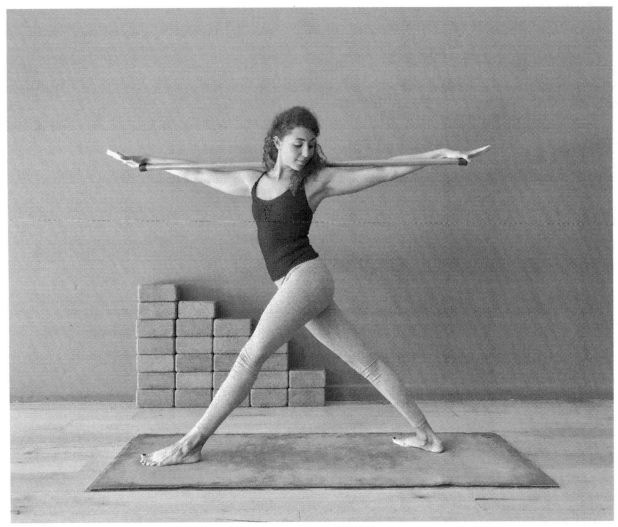

Side view

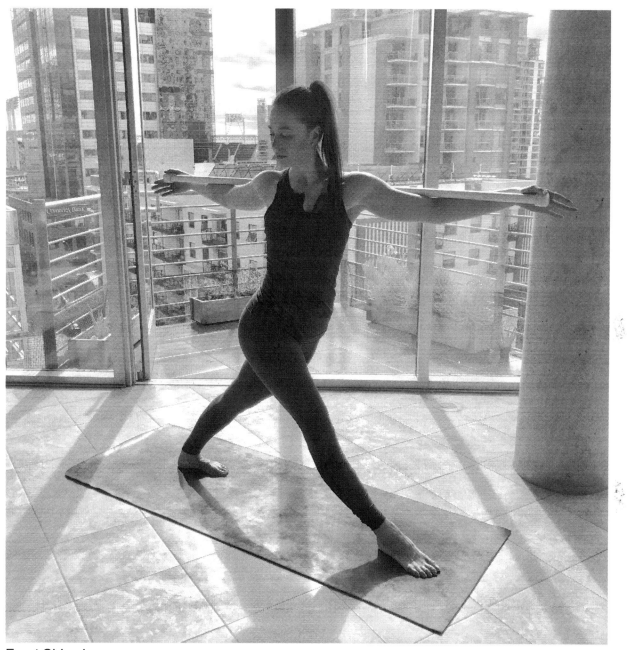

Front Side view

Eel

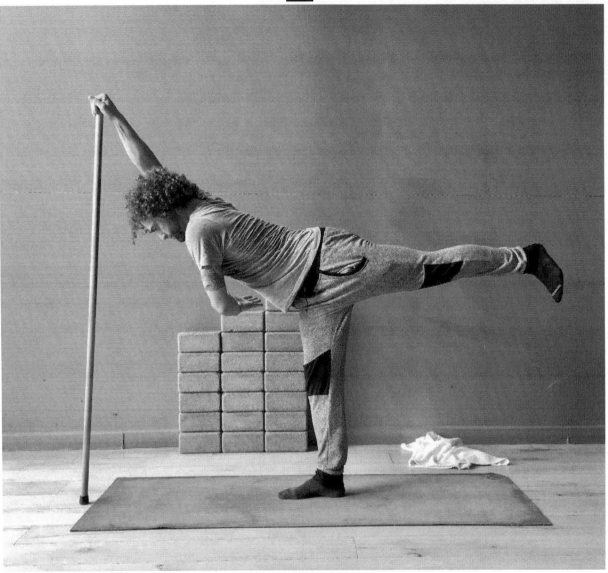

Side view

Elephant

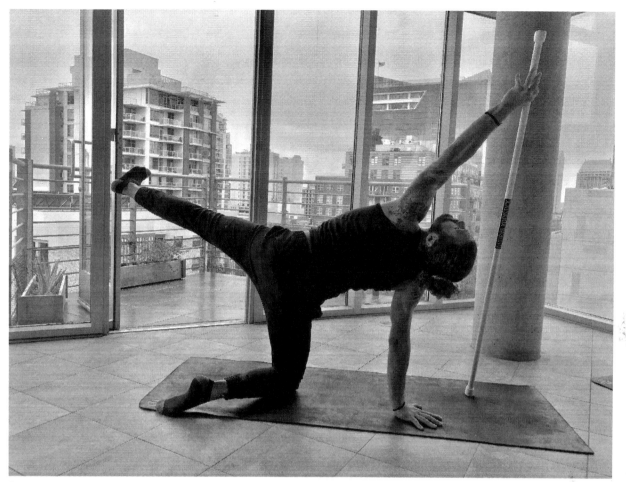

Rear View

Elevate

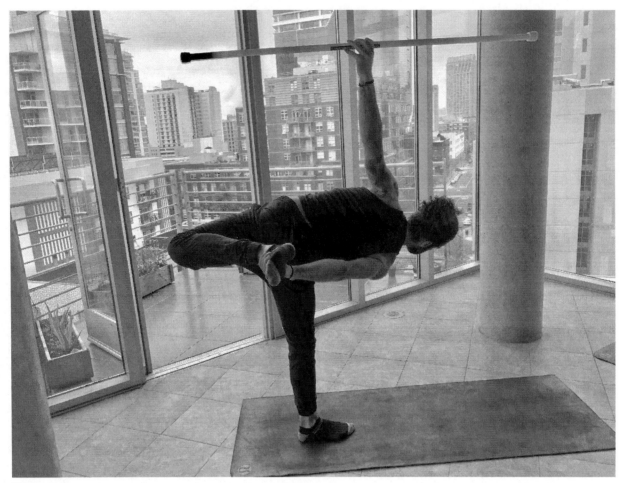

Rear view

Eskimo

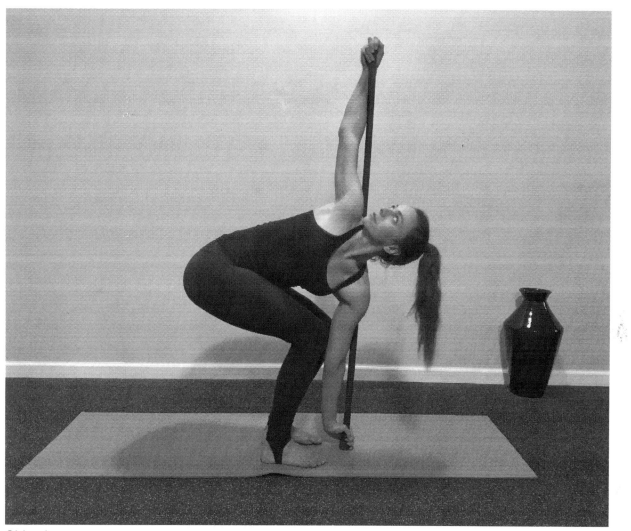
Side view

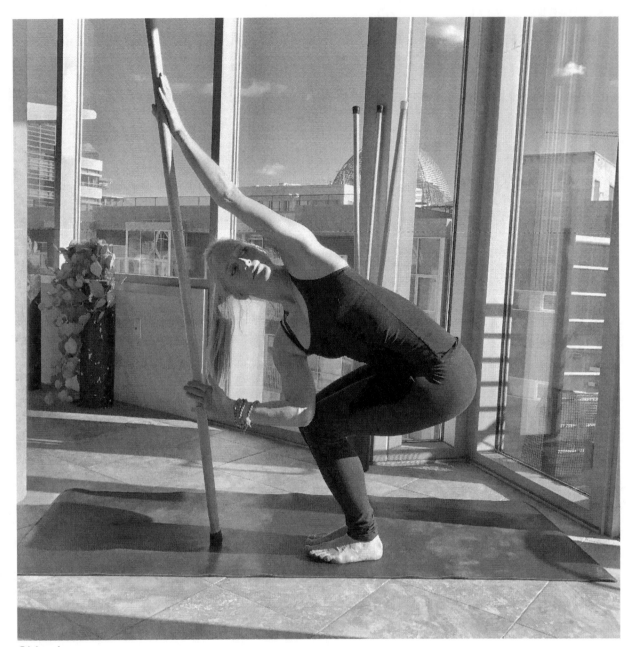

Side view

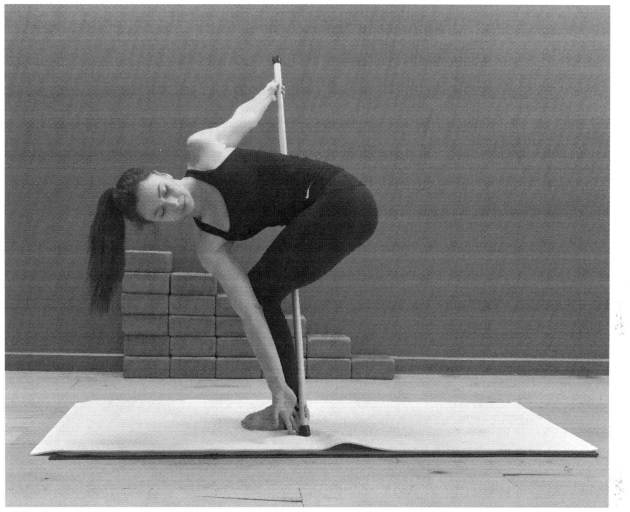

Side View

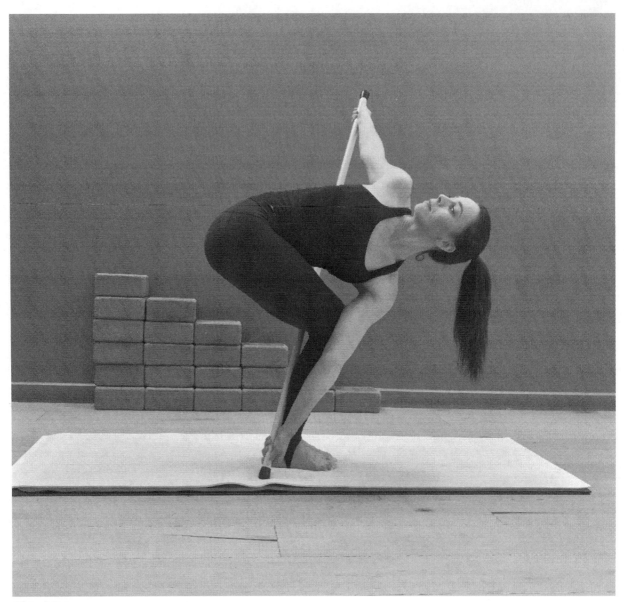

Side View

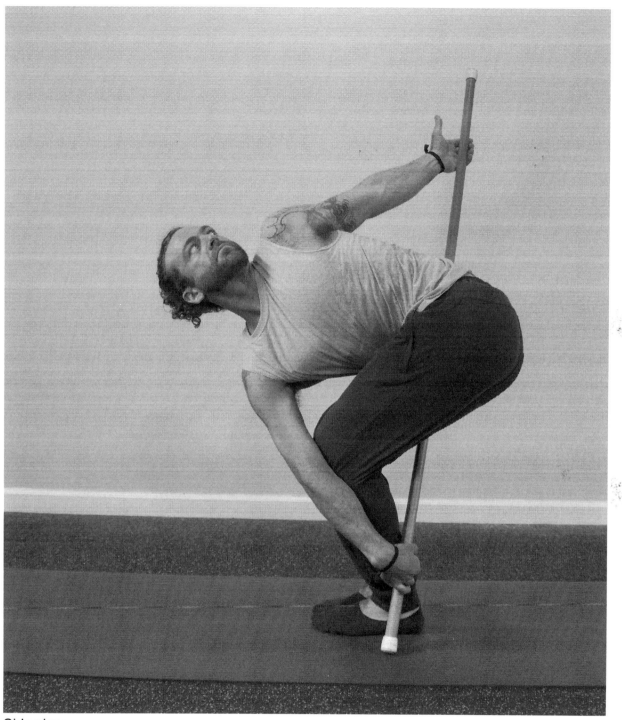

Side view

Evolve

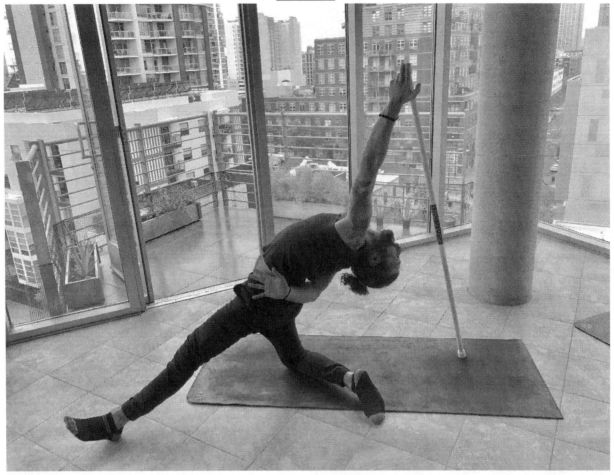

Side Rear view

Evolved Star

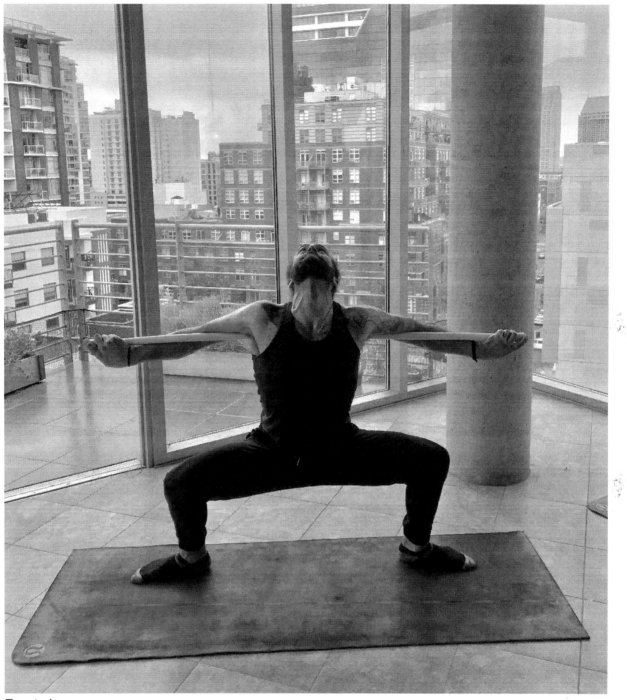

Front view

Extended Side Angle

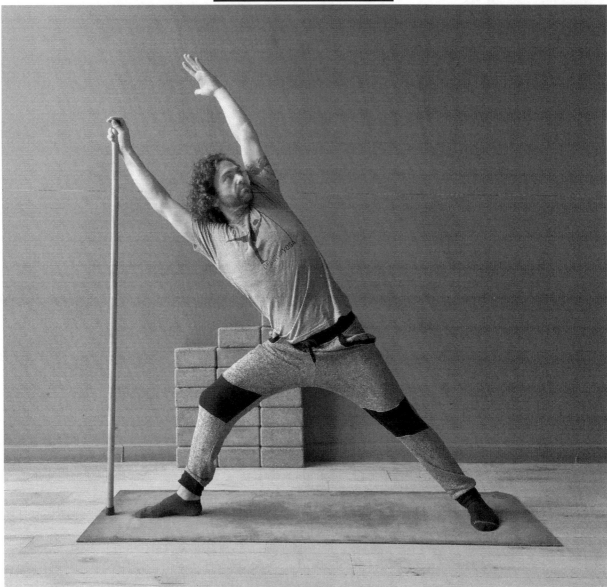

Front view

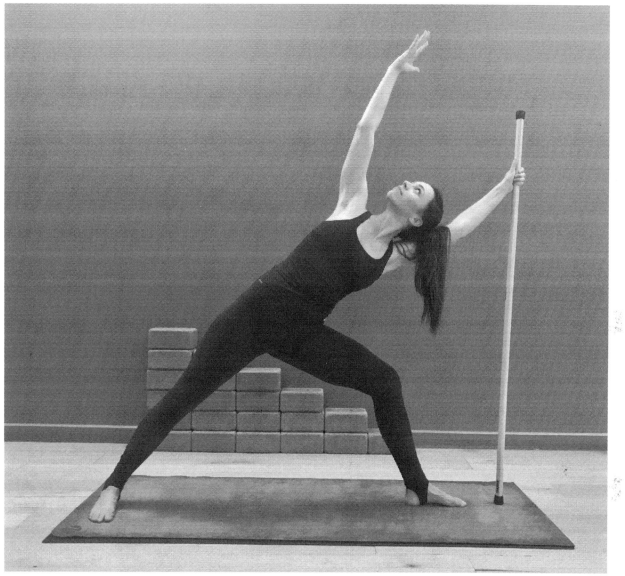

Side view

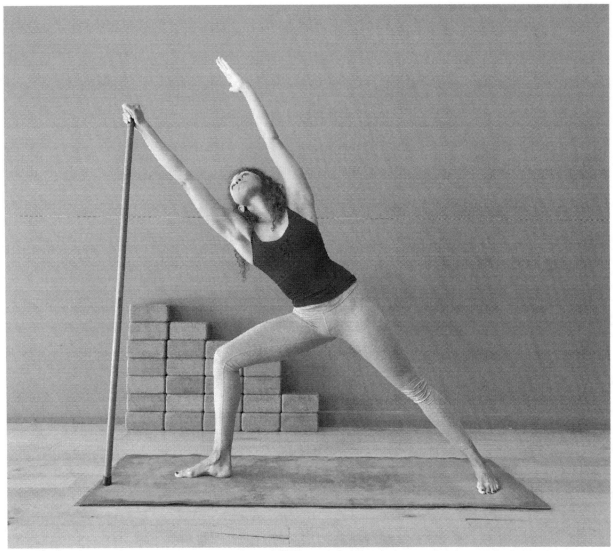

Side view

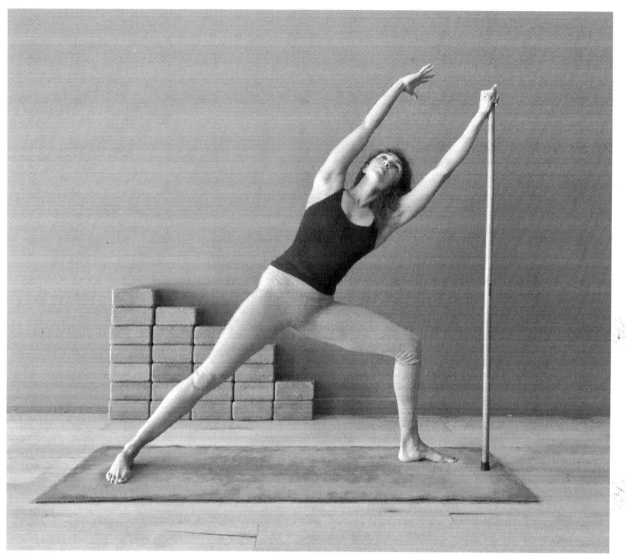
Side view

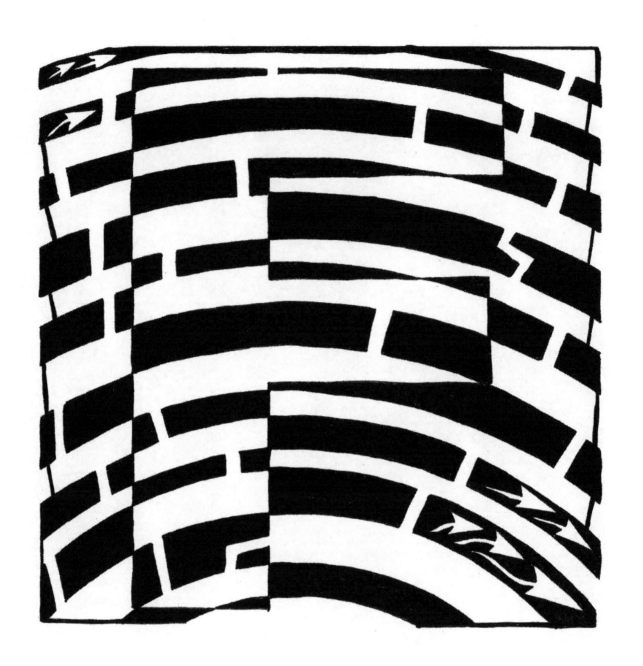

Falcon

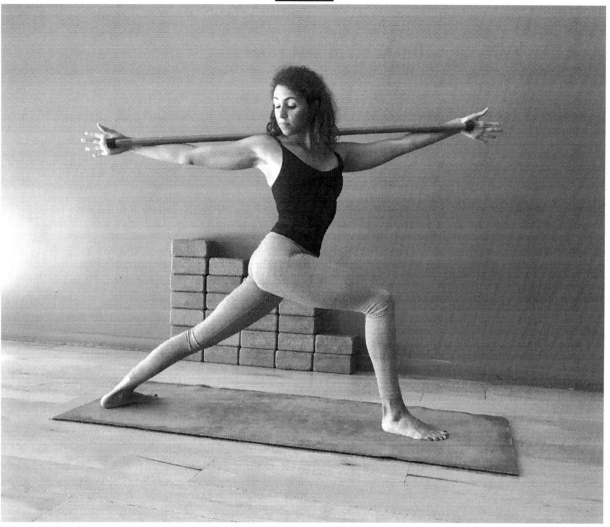

Front Side view

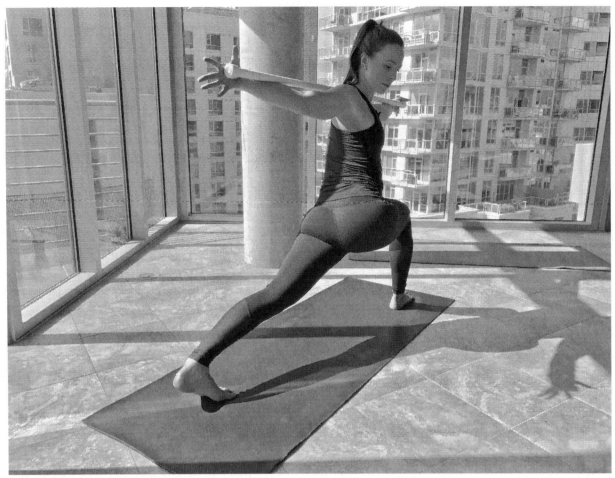

Rear Side view

Firefly

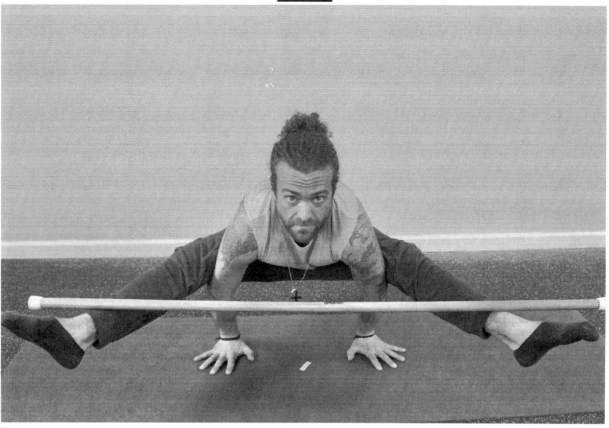

Front view

117

Fire

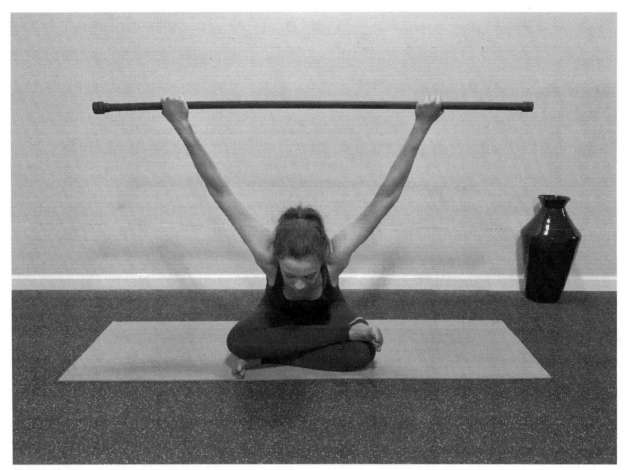
Front view

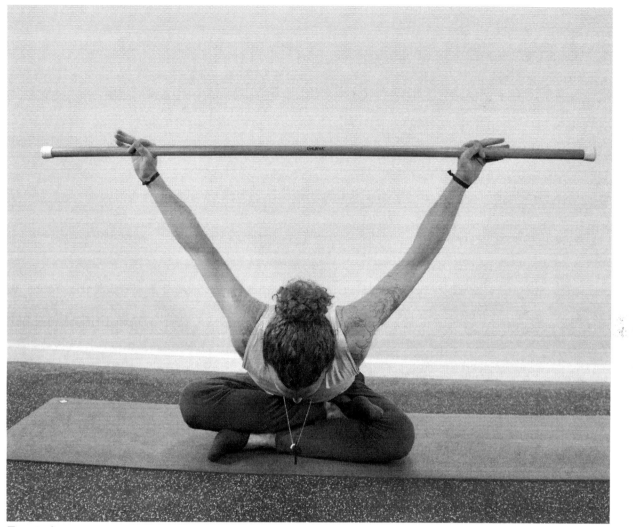
Front view

Fire Log

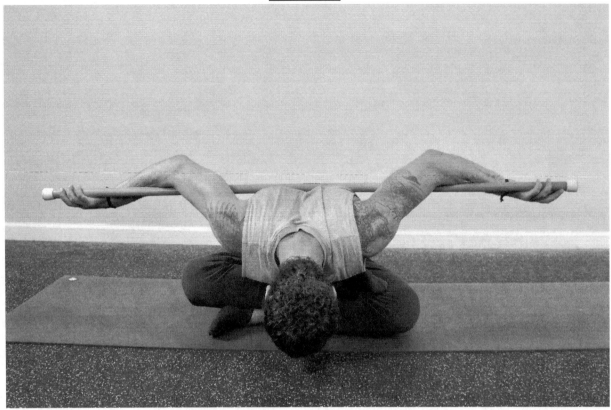

Front view

Fish

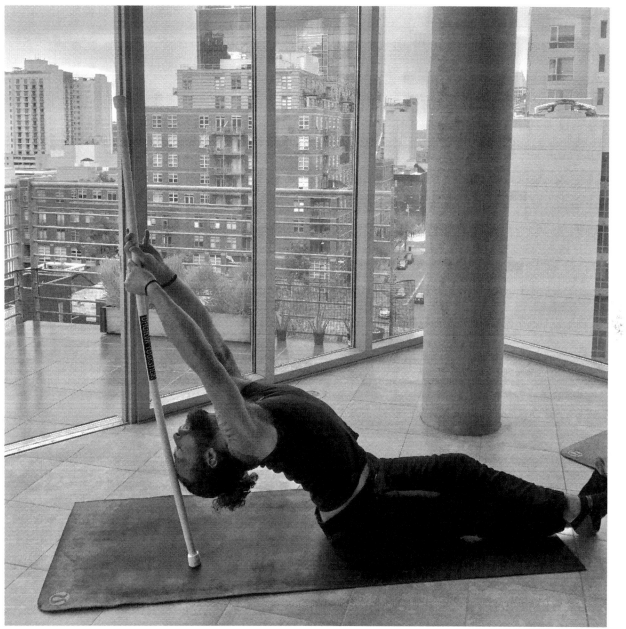

Side view

Flamingo

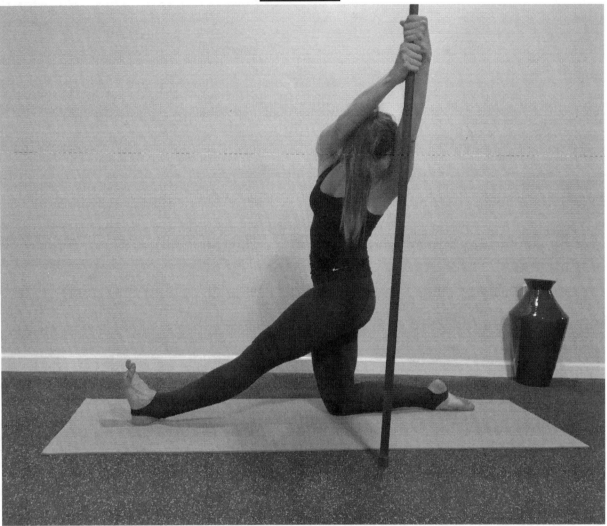

Side view

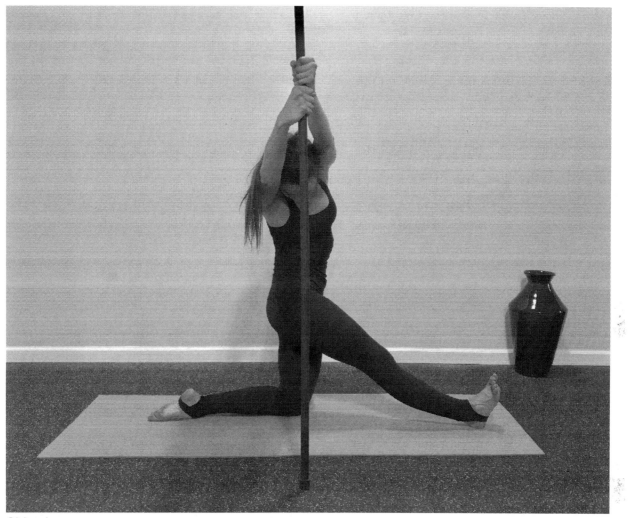
Side view

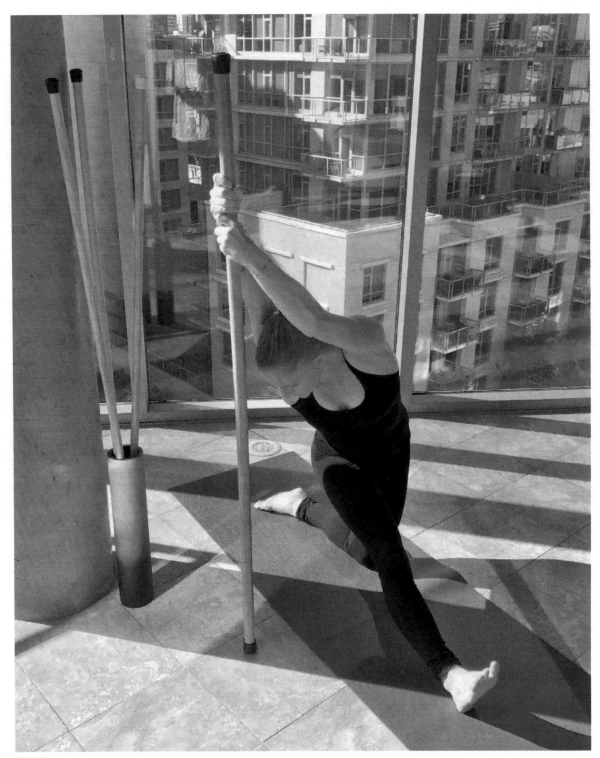

Front Side view

Flying Pigeon

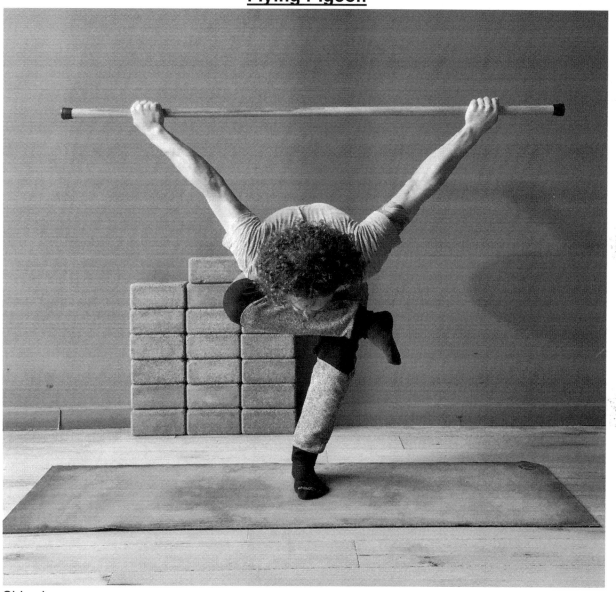

Side view

Flying Squirrel

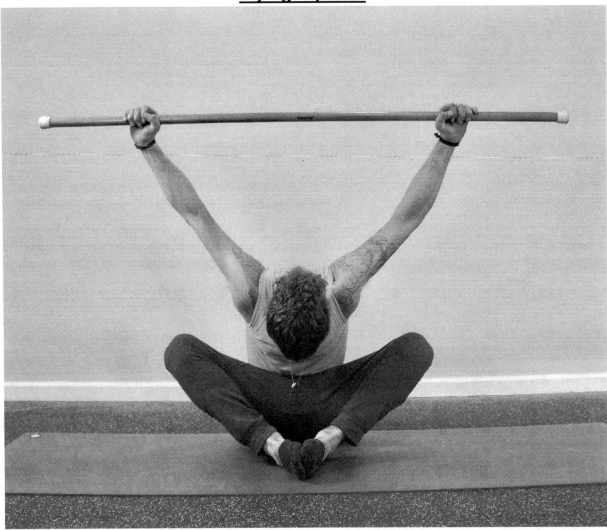

Front view

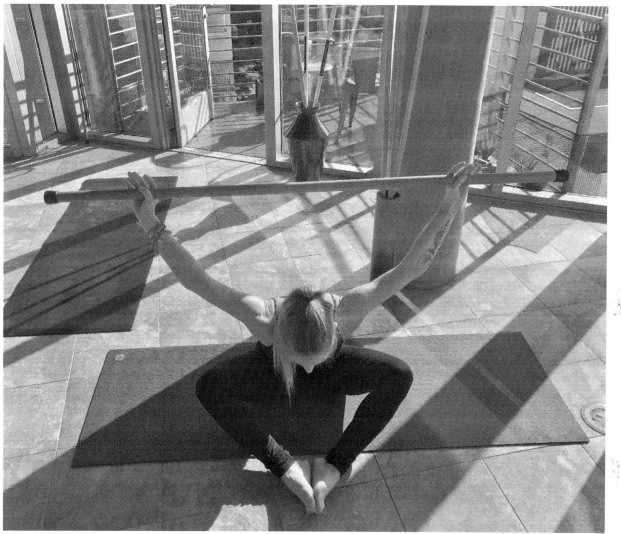

Front view

Forearm Side Plank

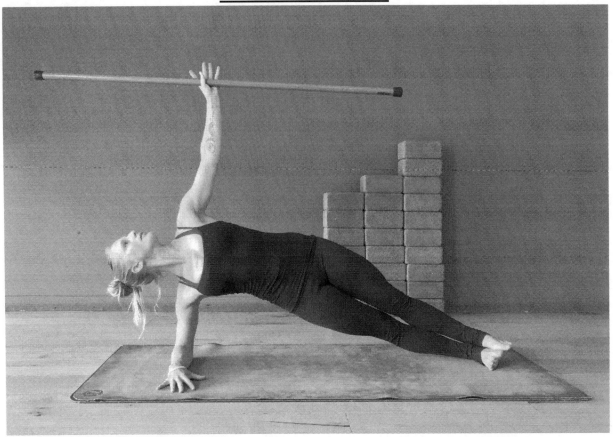

Front Side view

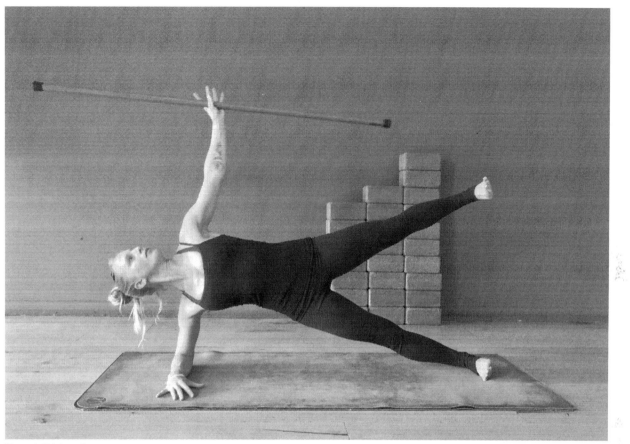
Front Side view

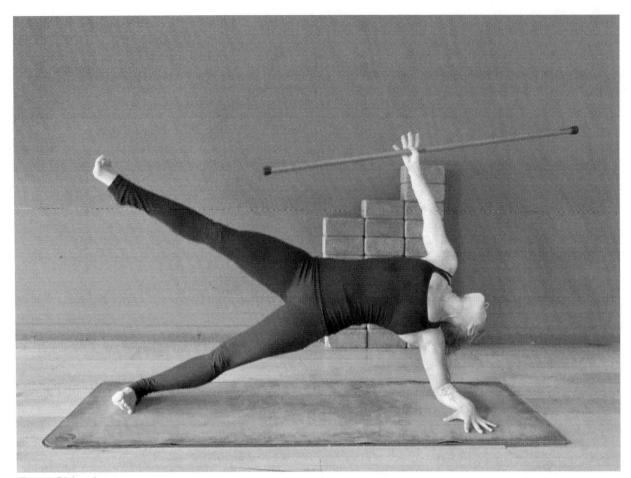

Front Side view

Freedom

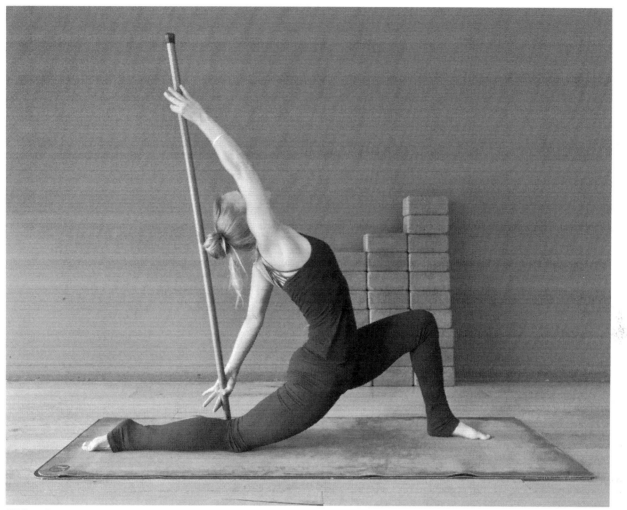
Side view

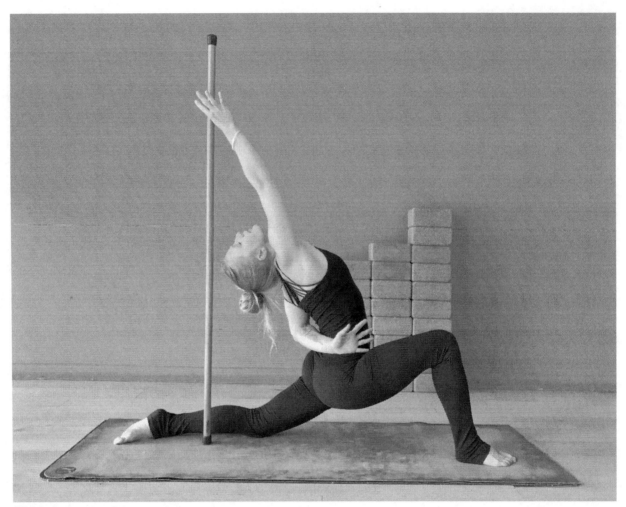

Side view

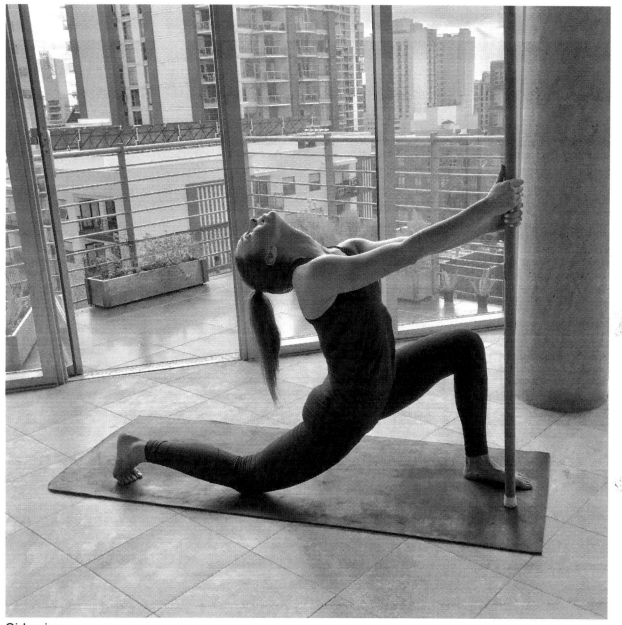

Side view

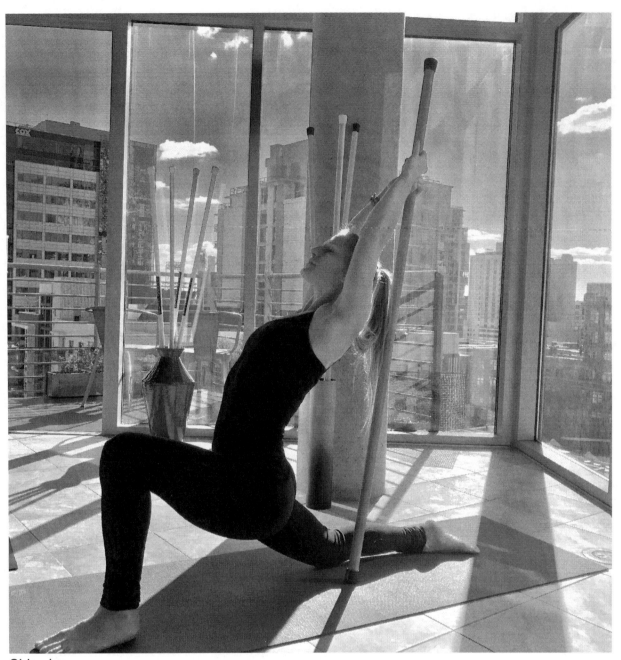
Side view

Full Moon

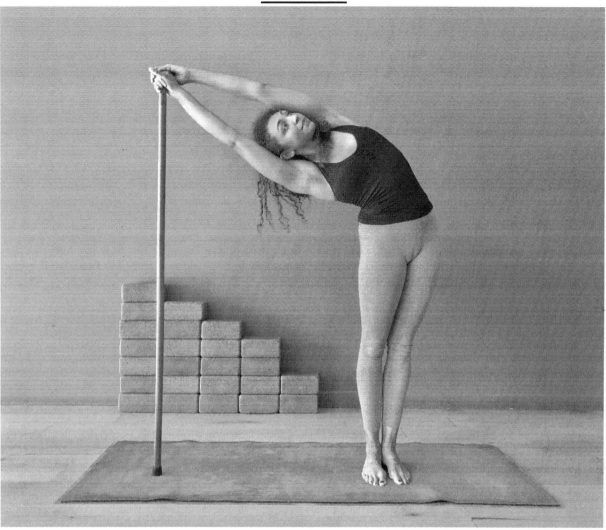

Front view

135

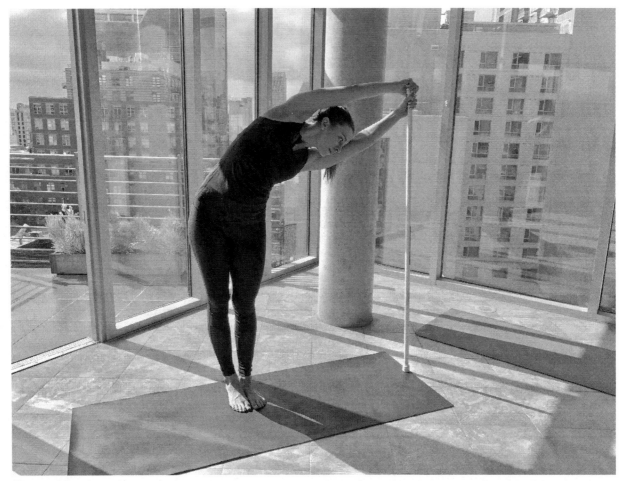

Front view

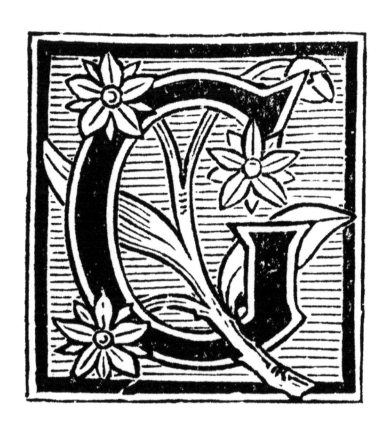

Gate

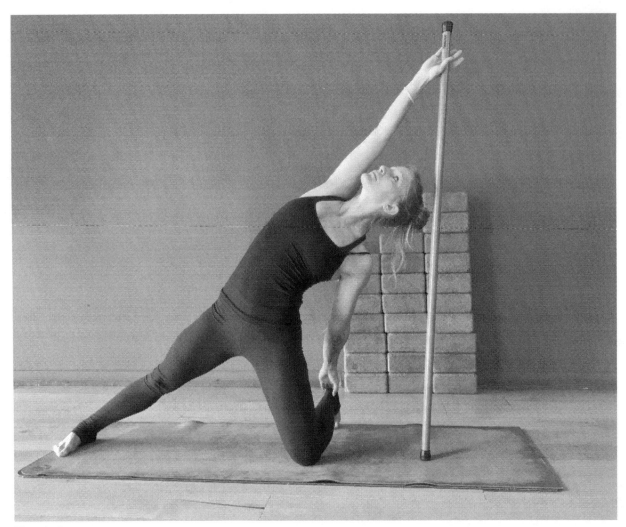

Front view

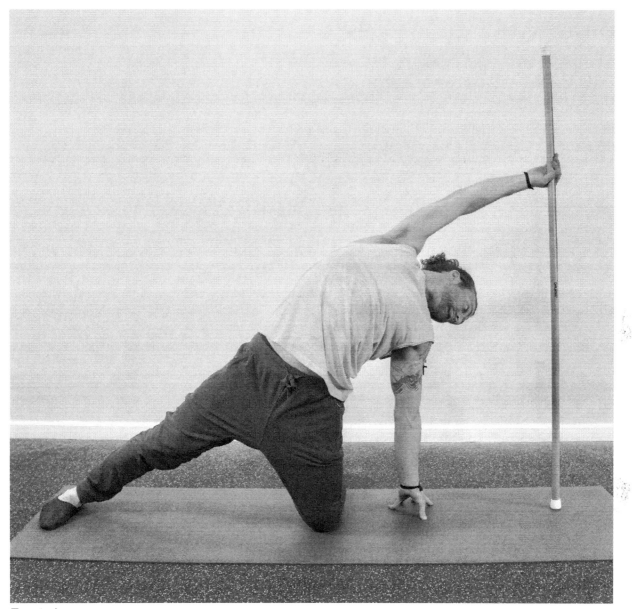

Front view

Gemini

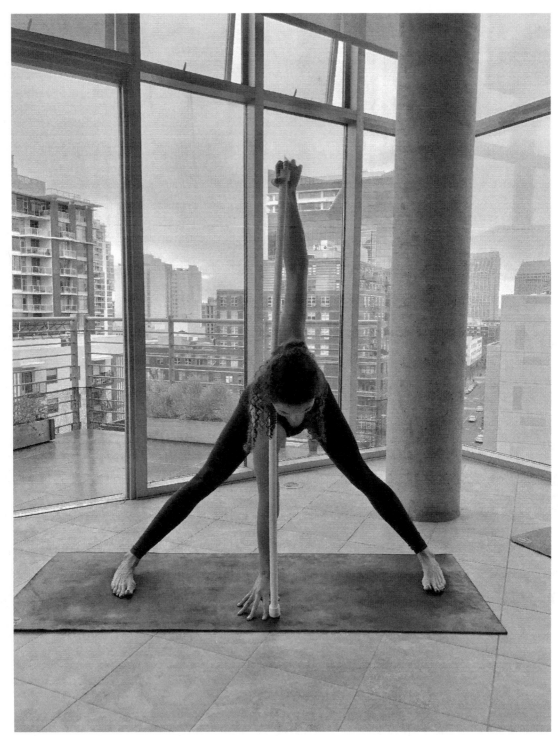

Front view

Giraffe

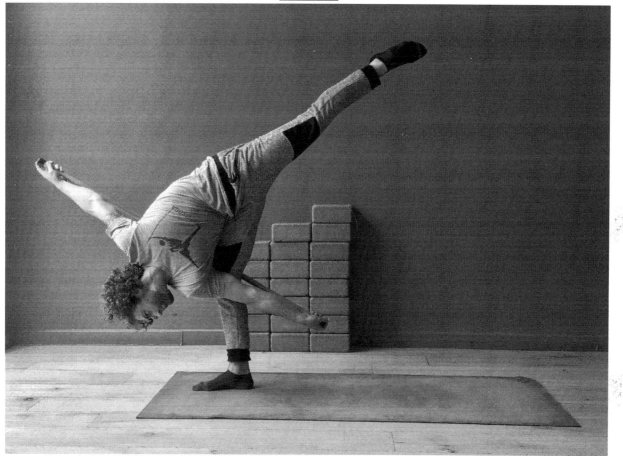

Side view

Glacier

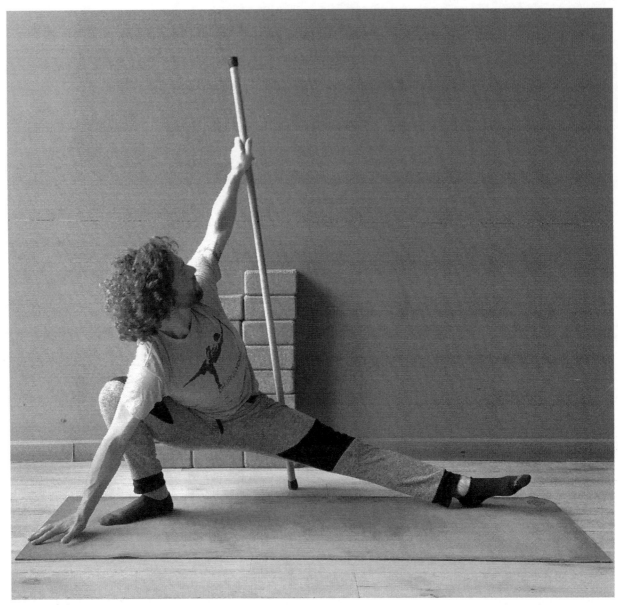

Front view

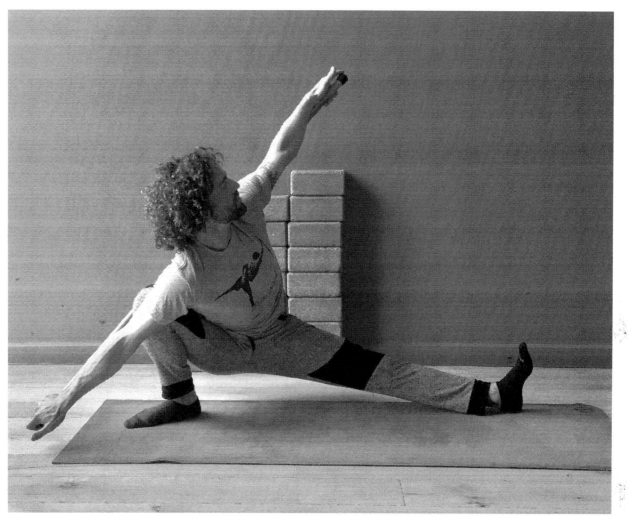
Front view

143

Goat

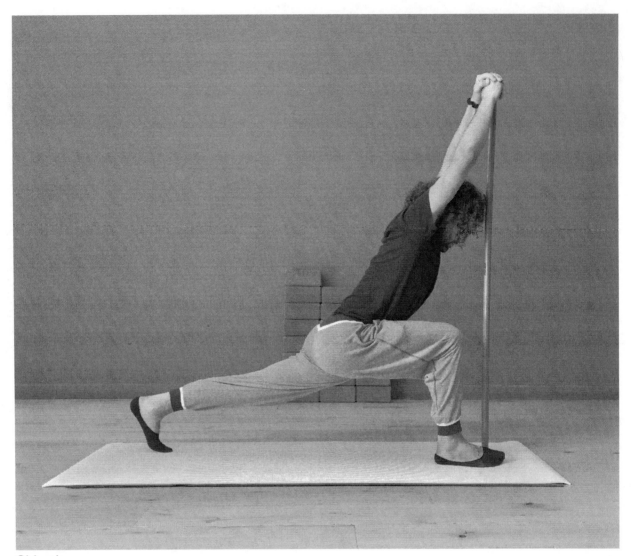
Side view

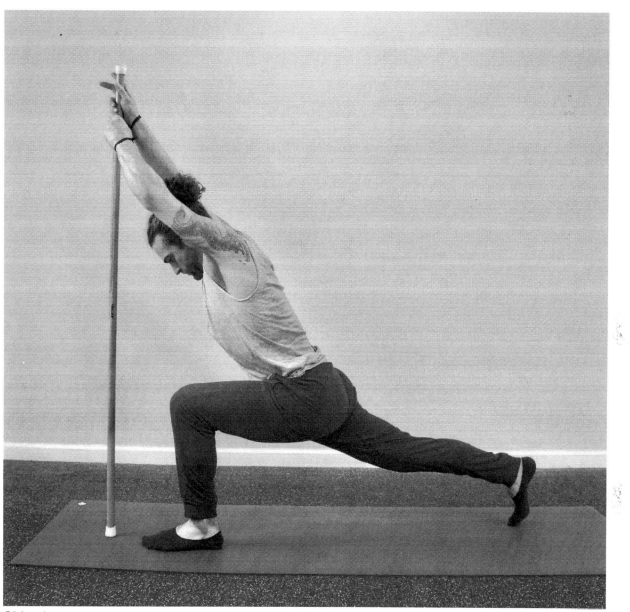

Side view

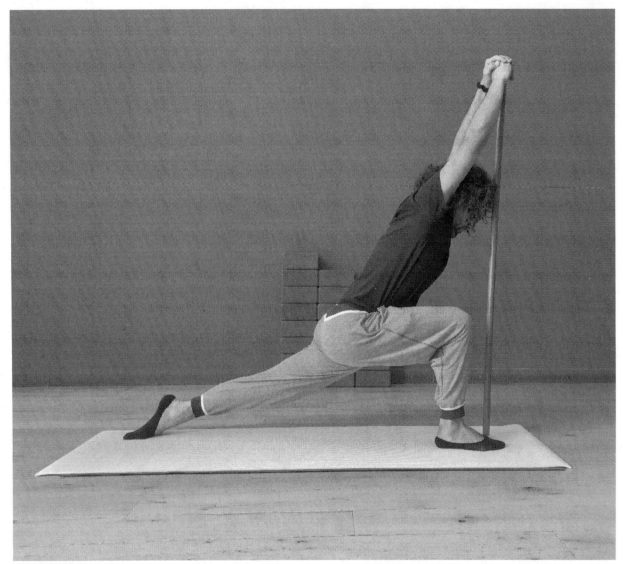
Side view

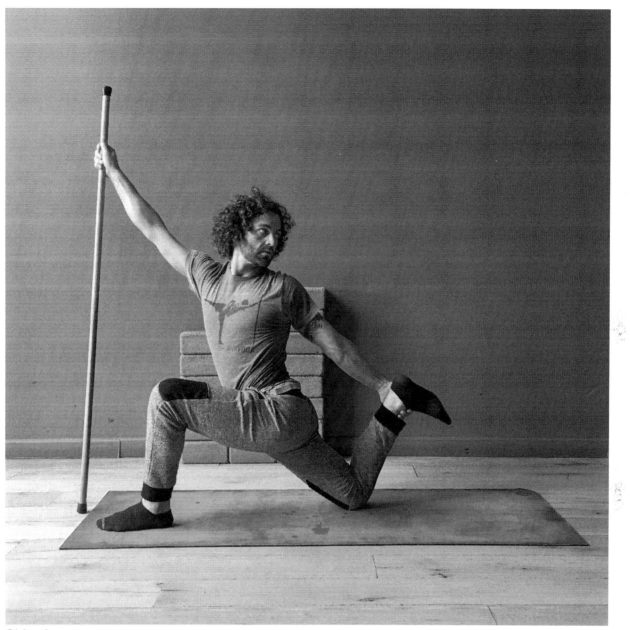

Side view

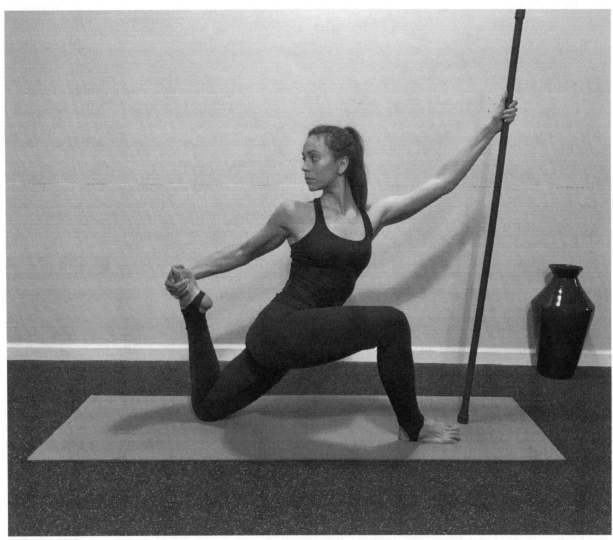
Side view

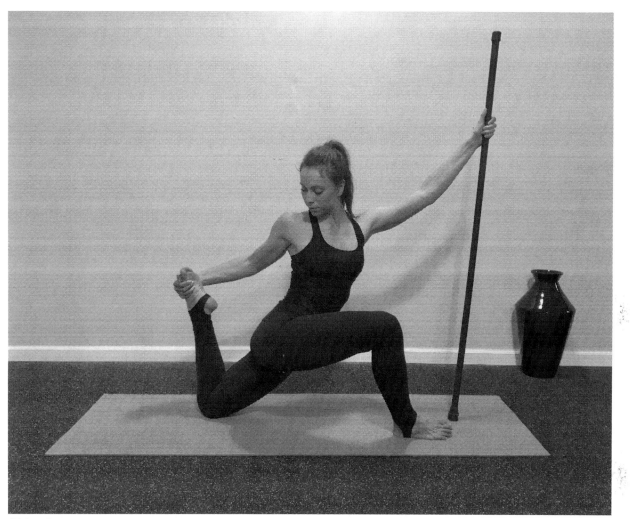

Side view

Gratitude

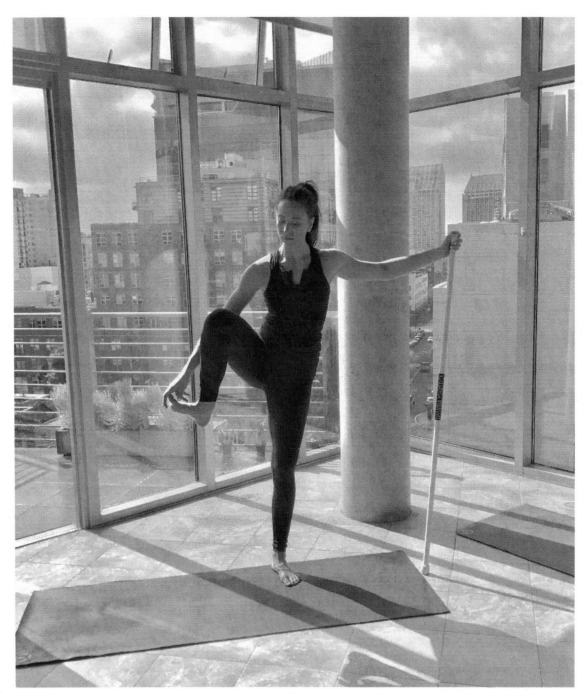

Front view

Great Wall

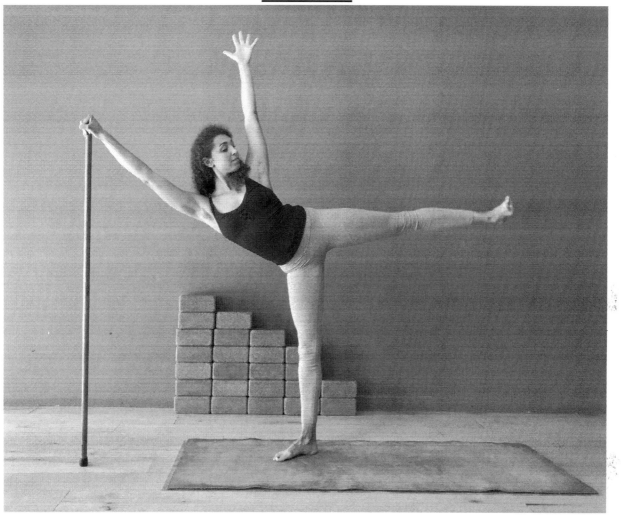

Front view

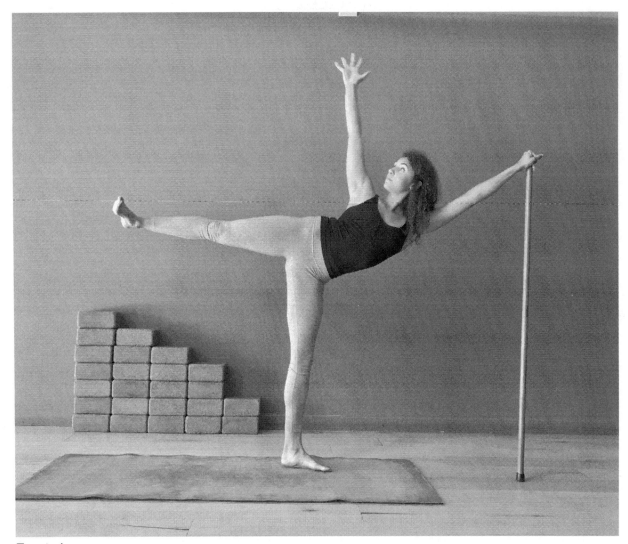

Front view

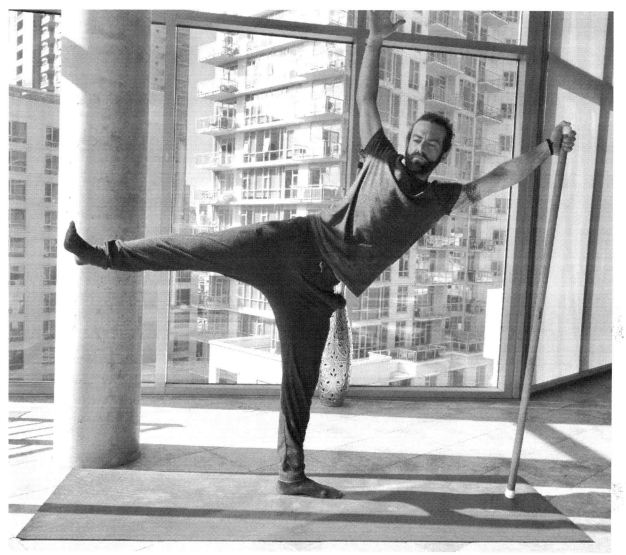

Front view

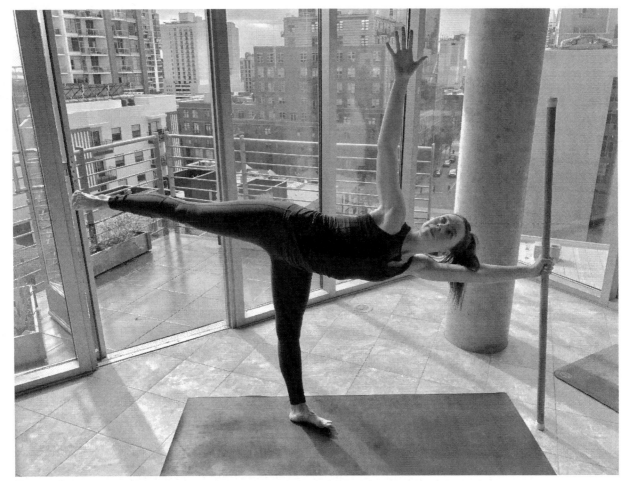
Front view

<u>Gypsy</u>

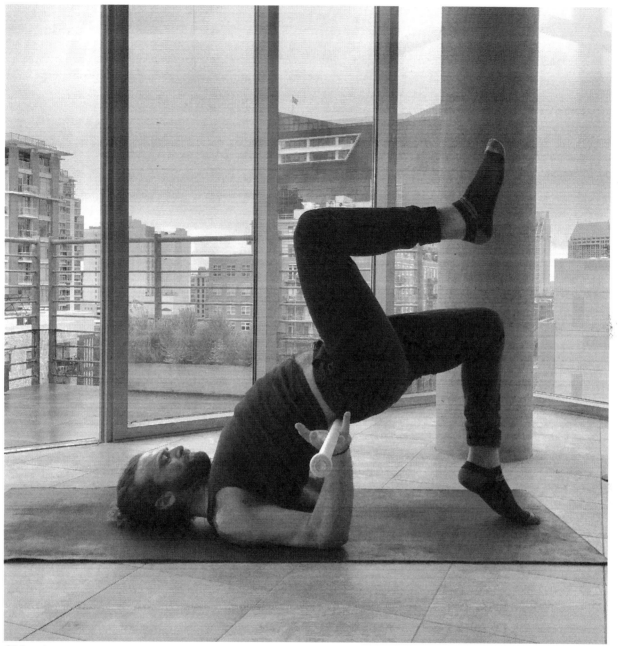

Side view

Gypsy Soul

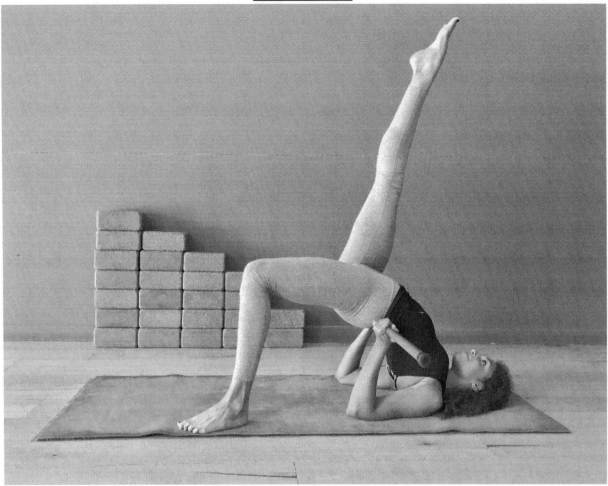

Side view

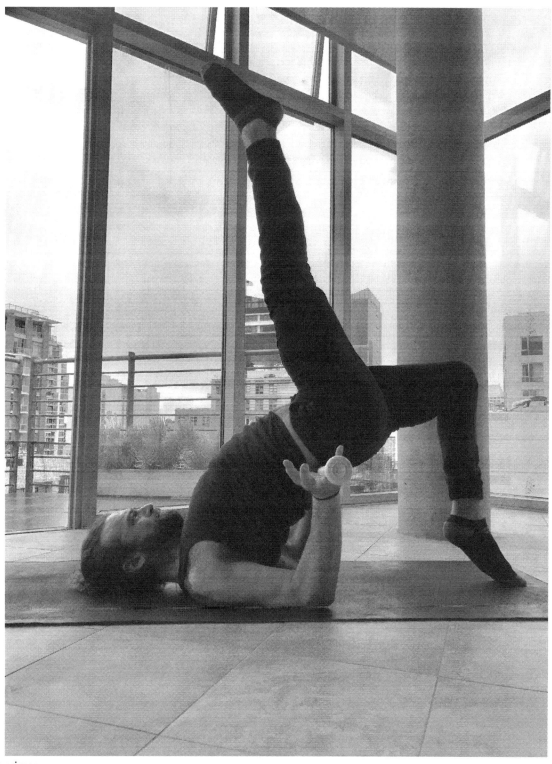

Side view

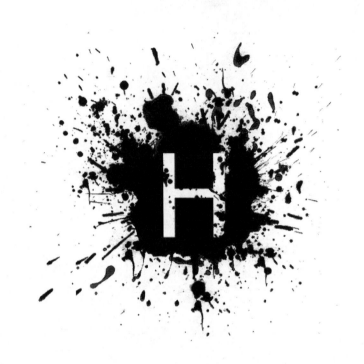

Halfway Lift

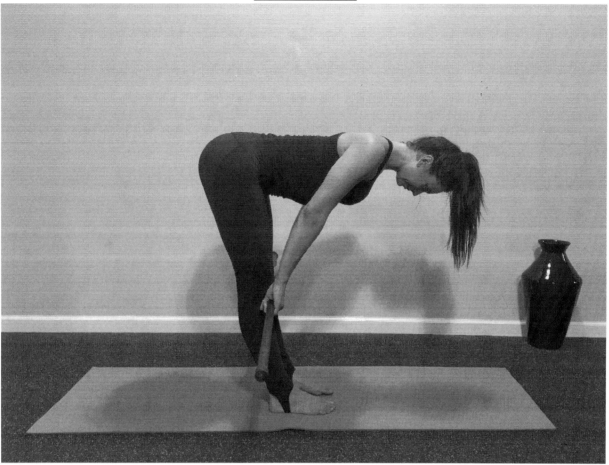

Side view

Half Moon

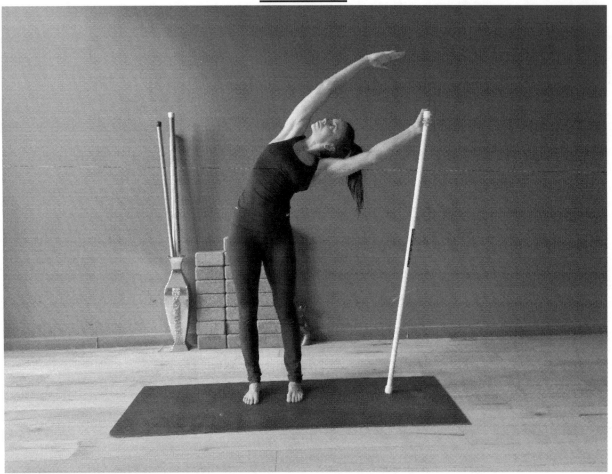

Front view

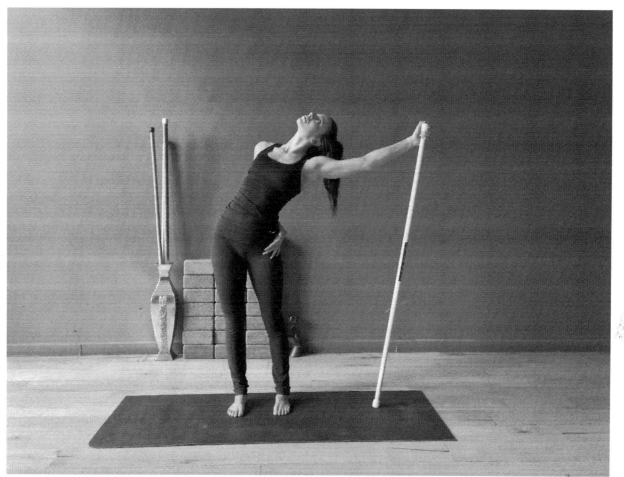

Front view

161

__Half Splits__

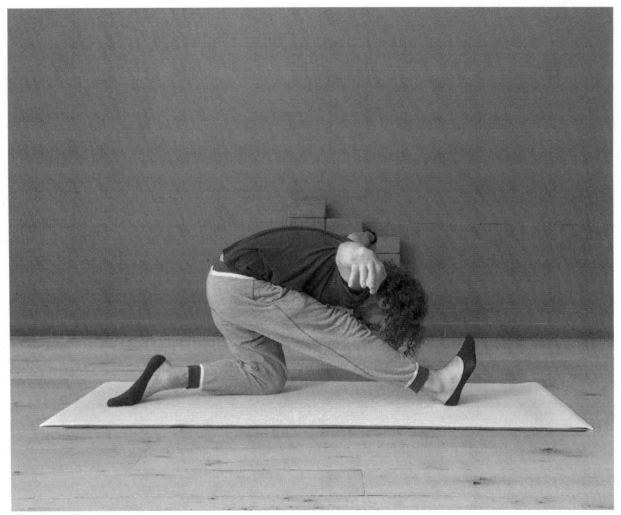
Side view

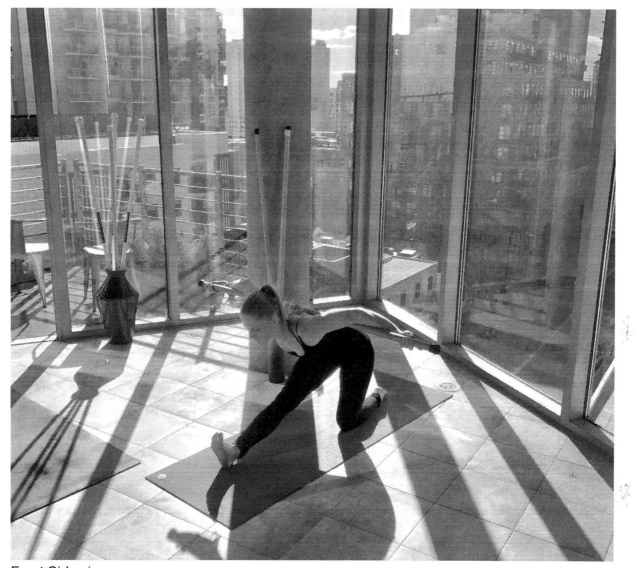

Front Side view

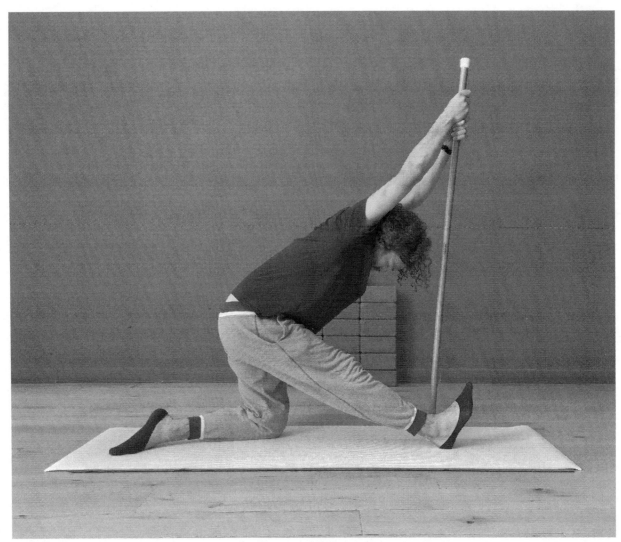

Side view

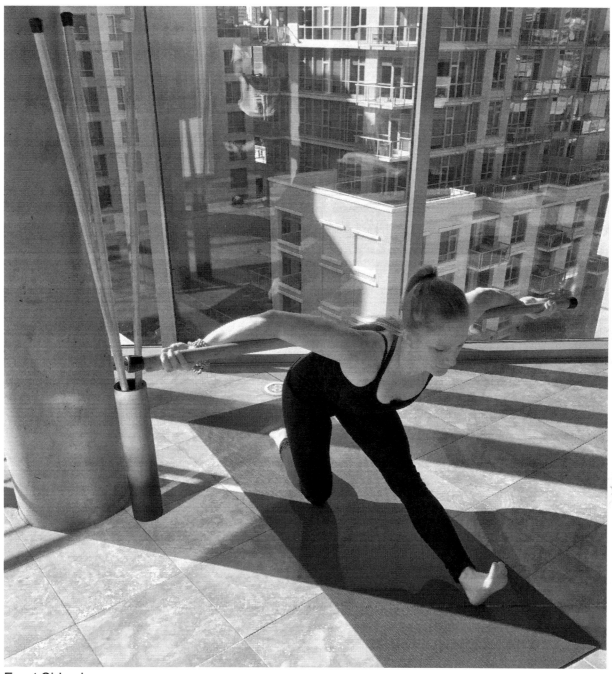

Front Side view

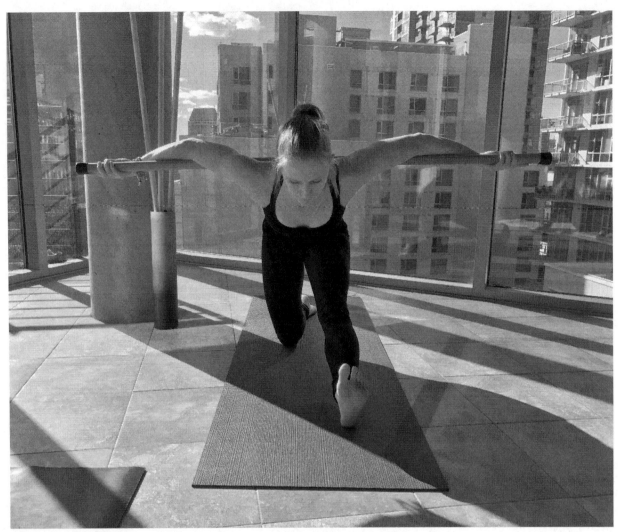

Front view

Happy Baby

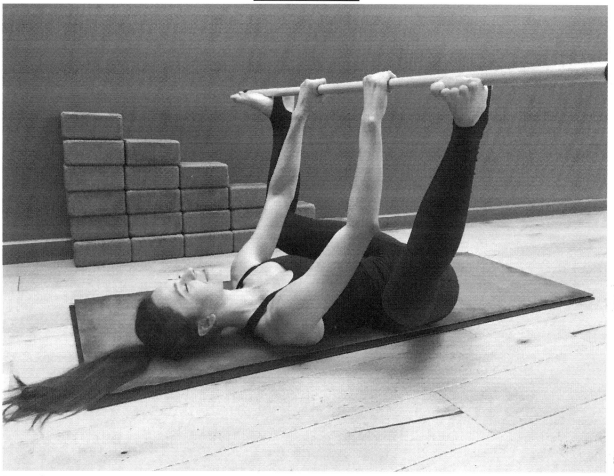

Rear Side View

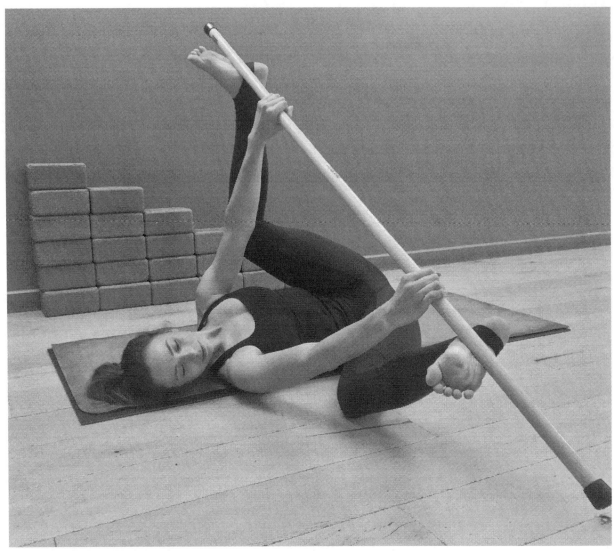

Rear Side View

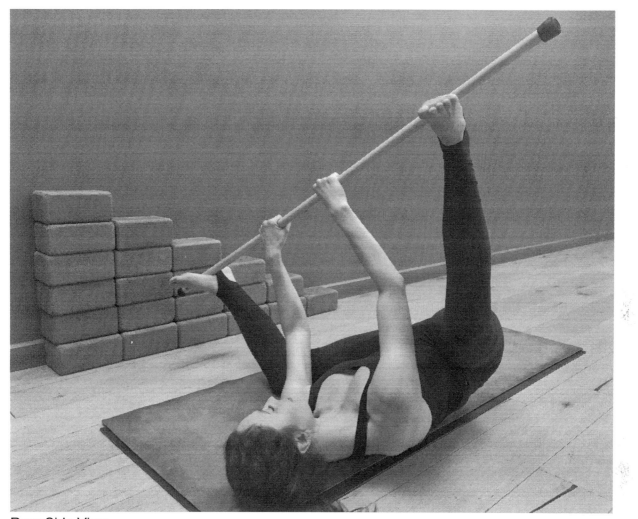

Rear Side View

169

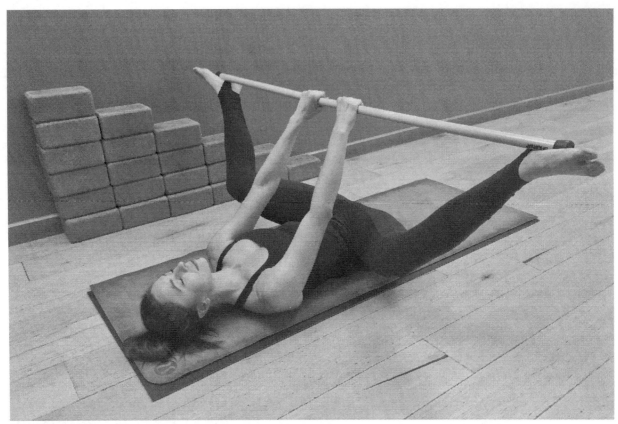

Rear Side View

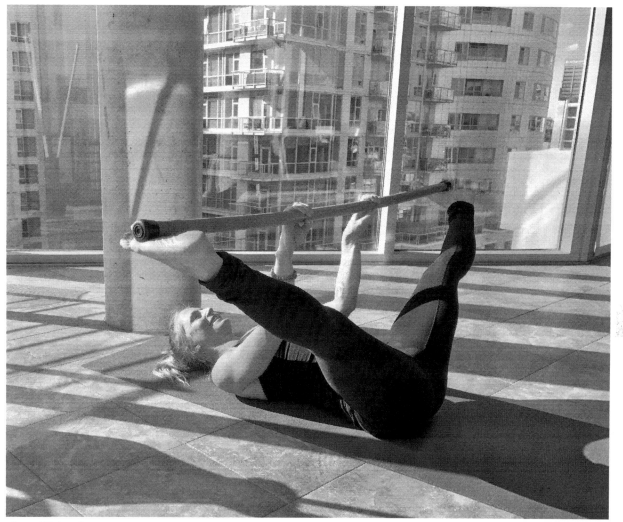
Rear Side view

Harry Potter

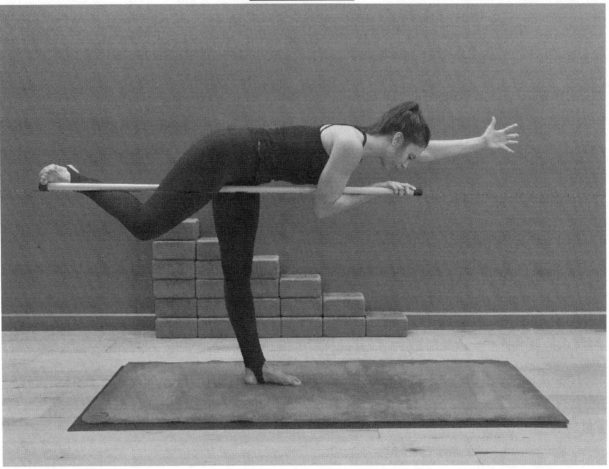

Side View

172

High Lunge

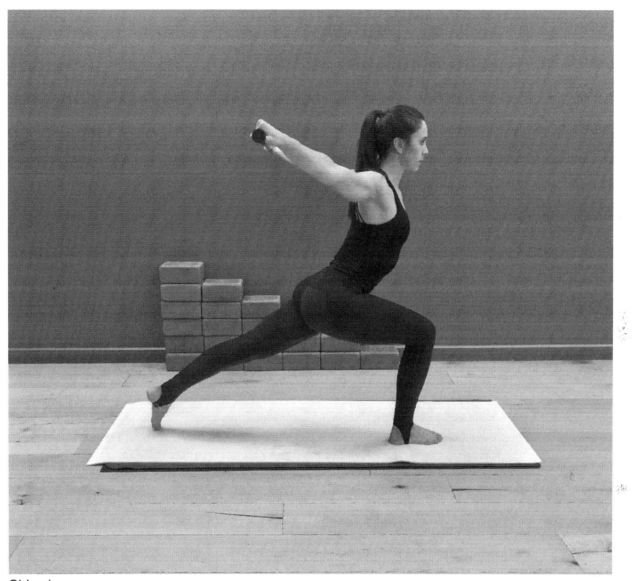

Side view

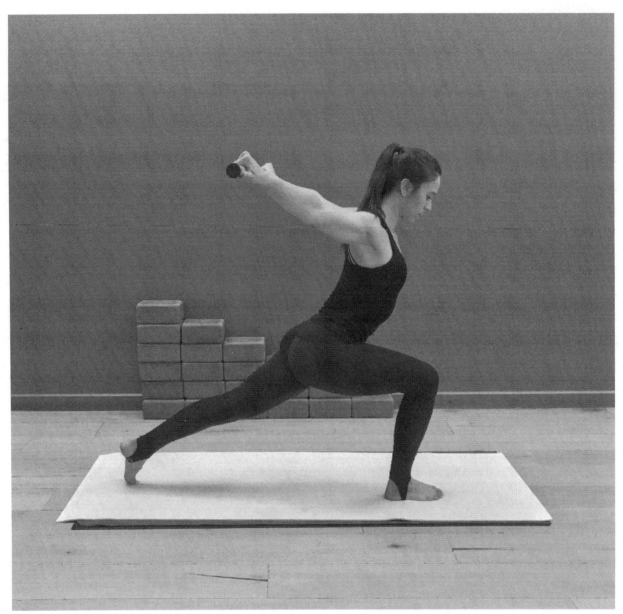
Side view

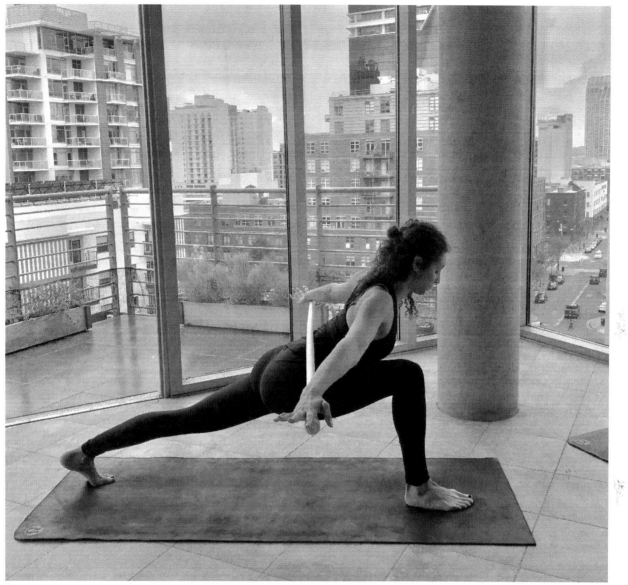
Side view

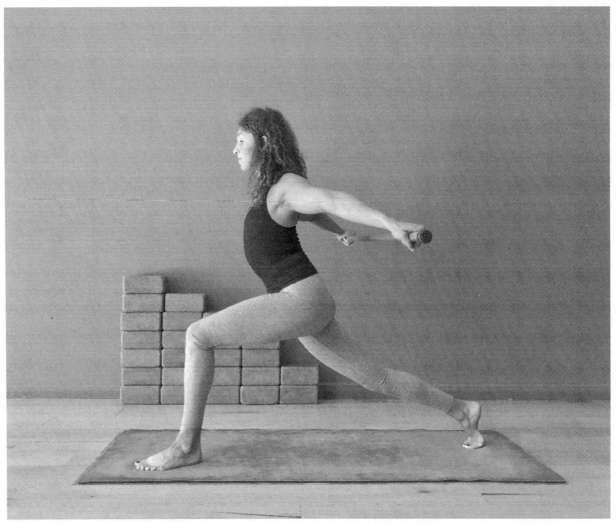
Side view

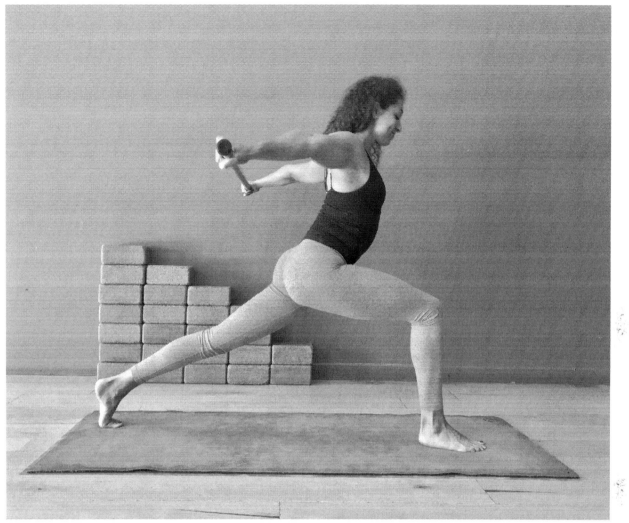

Side view

Horse

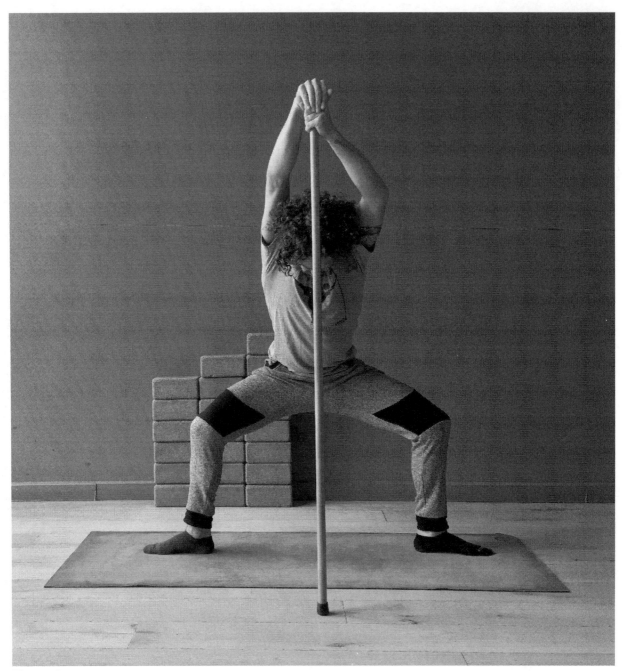

Front view

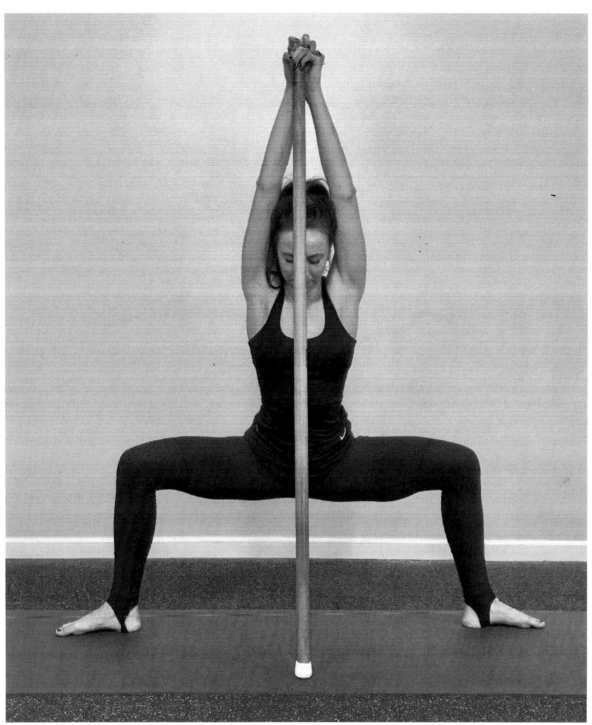

Front view

Humble Gypsy

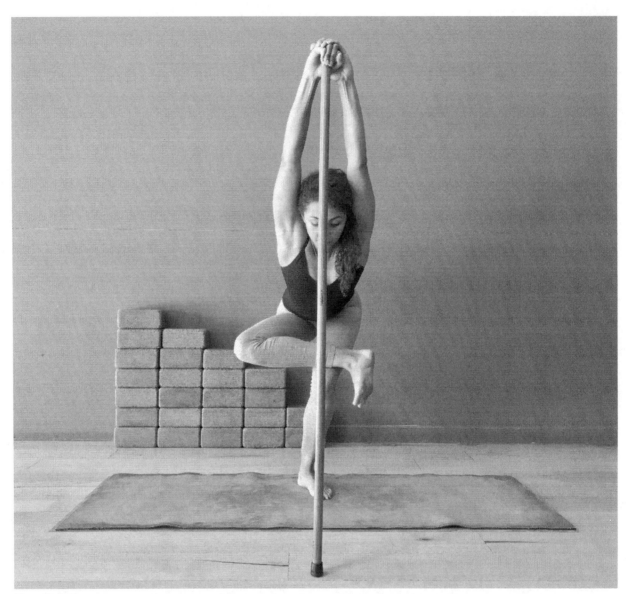

Front view

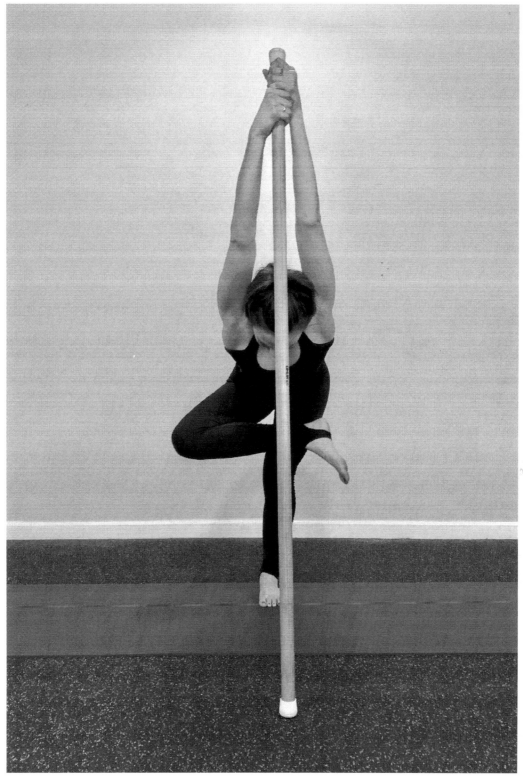

Front view

Humble Warrior

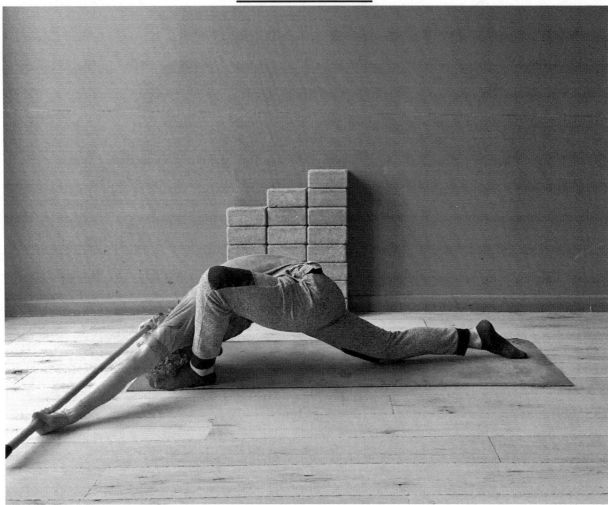

Side view

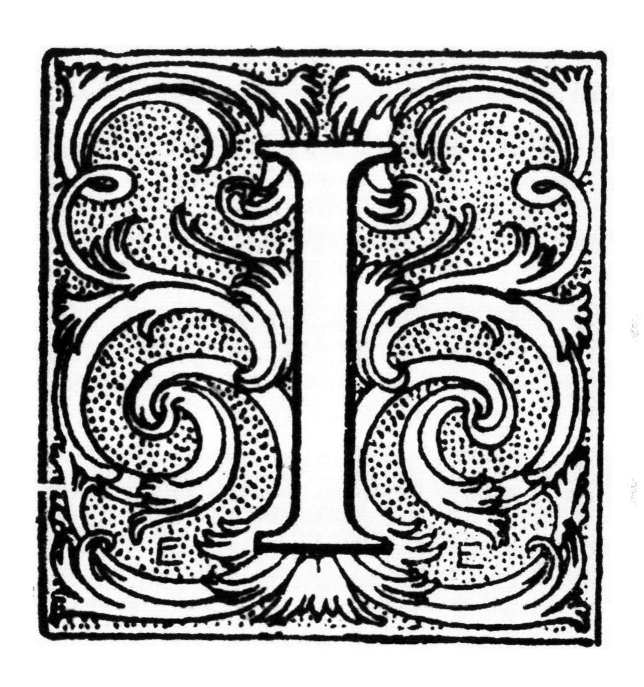

Impala

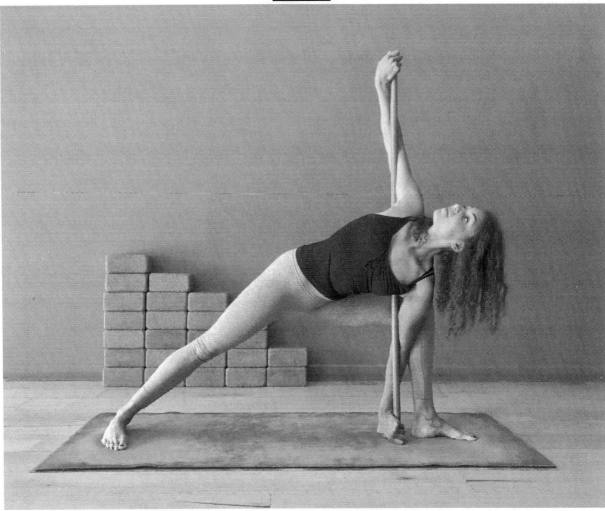

Front view

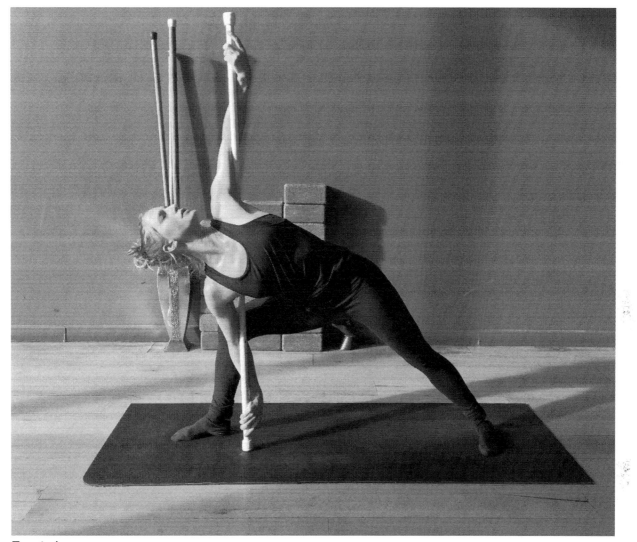
Front view

Inclination

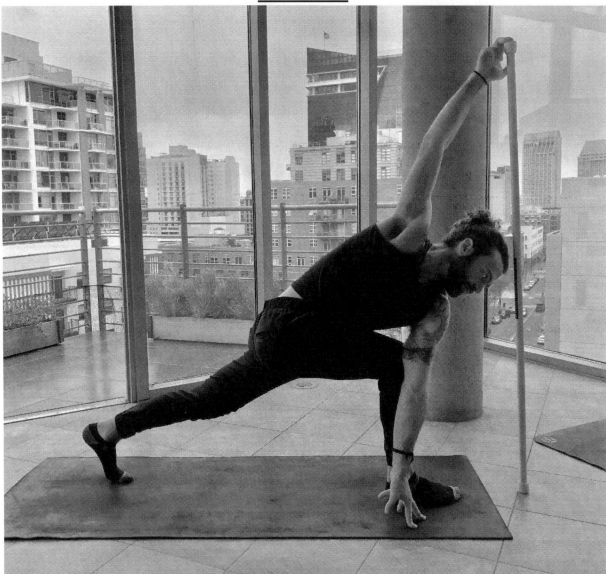

Side view

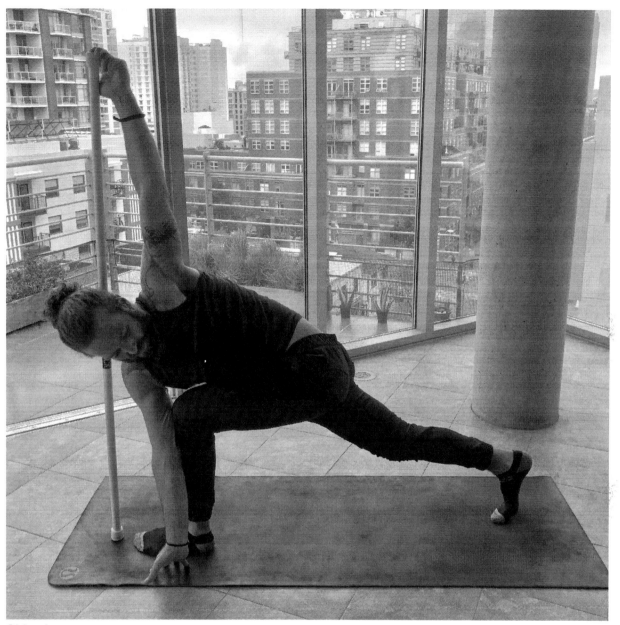

Side view

Indian Elephant

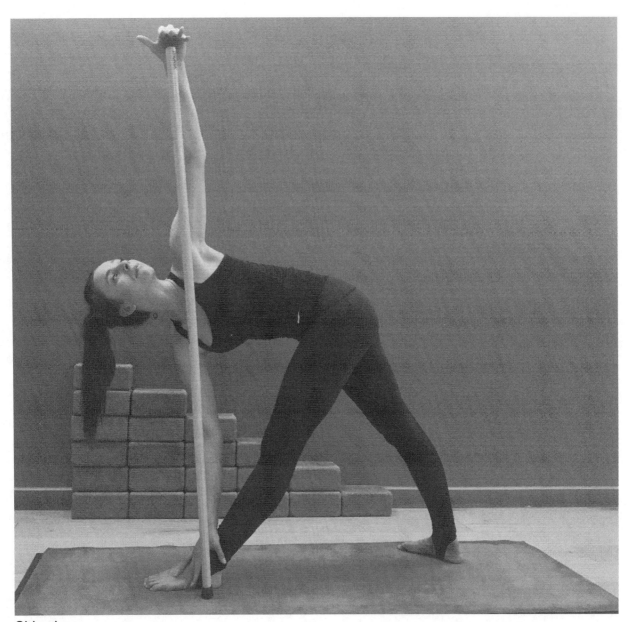

Side view

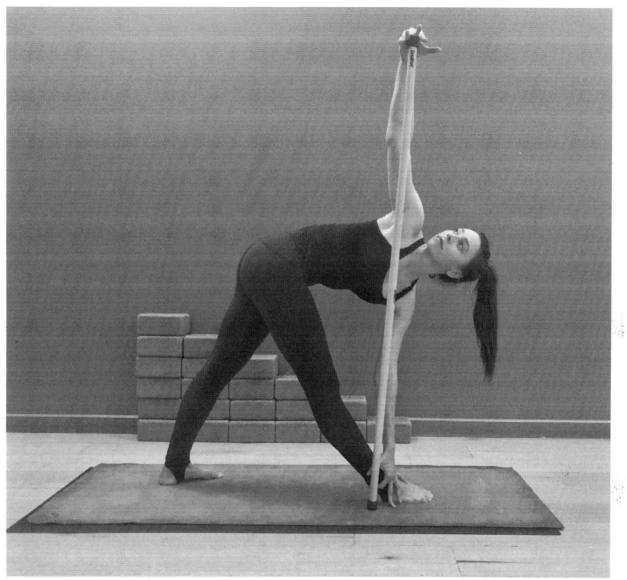

Side view

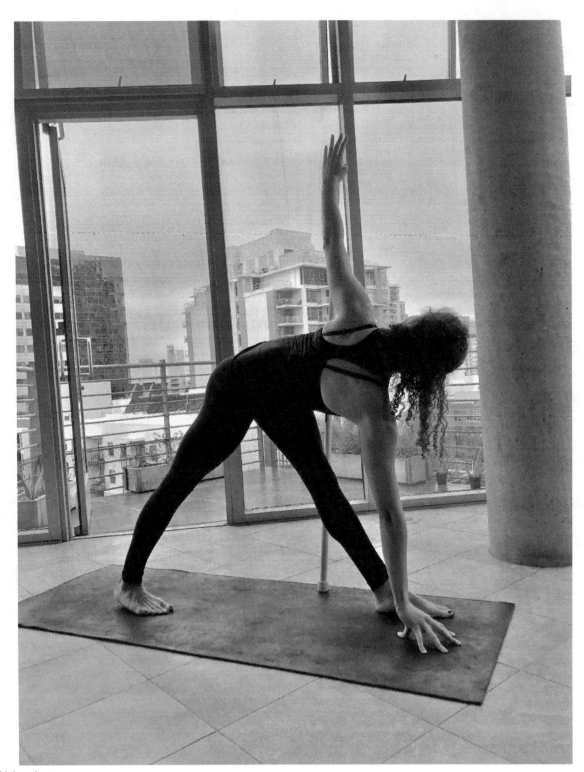

Side view

Inferno

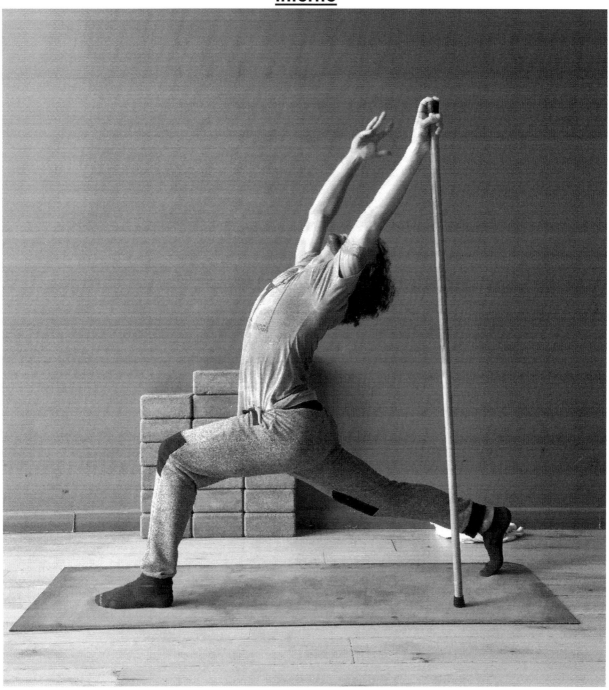

Side view

Intelligent

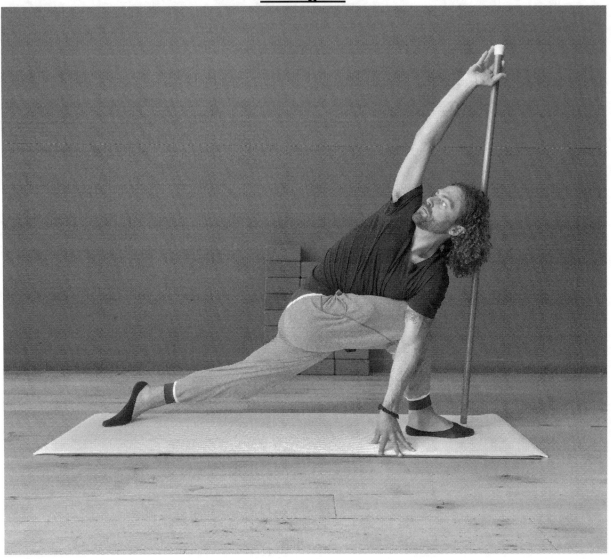

Side view

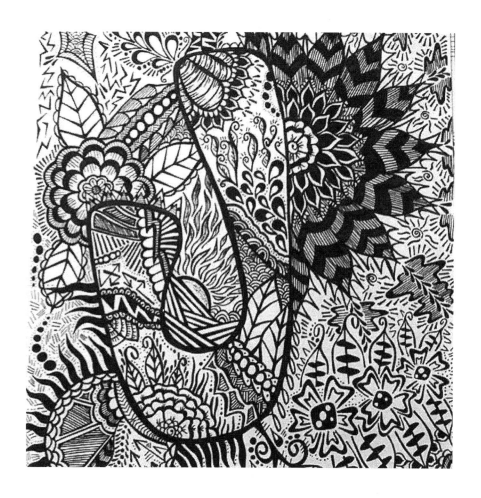

Javelin

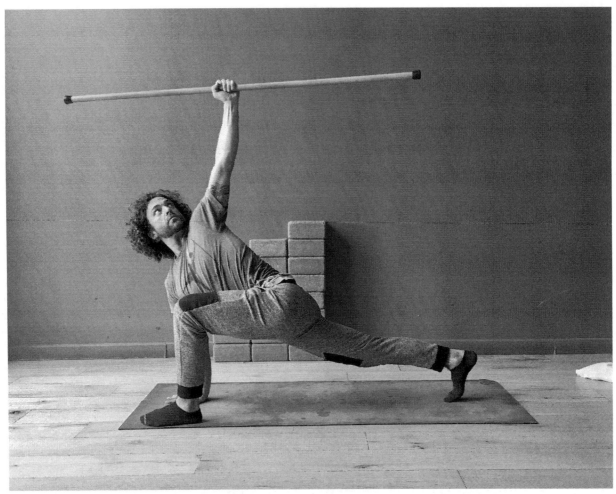

Side view

Juice

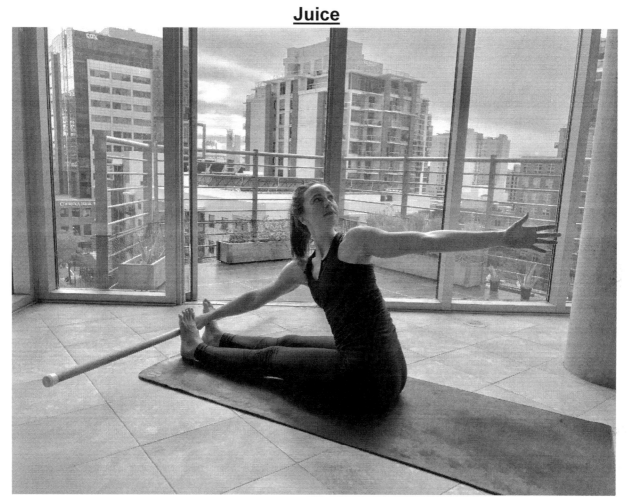

Side view

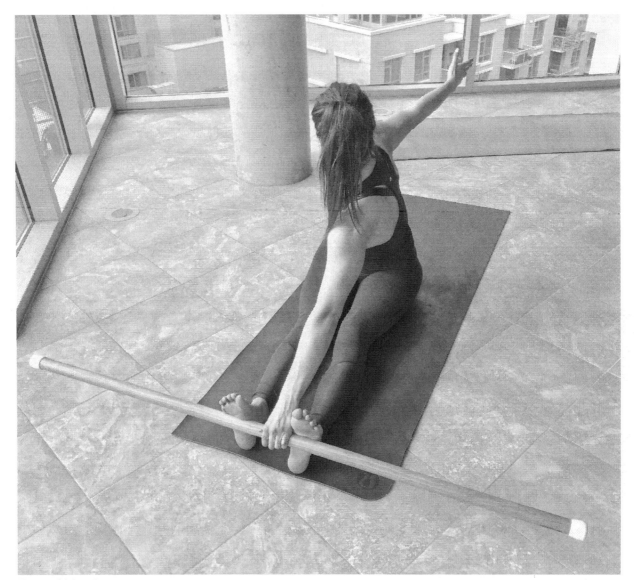

Front Side view

Juno

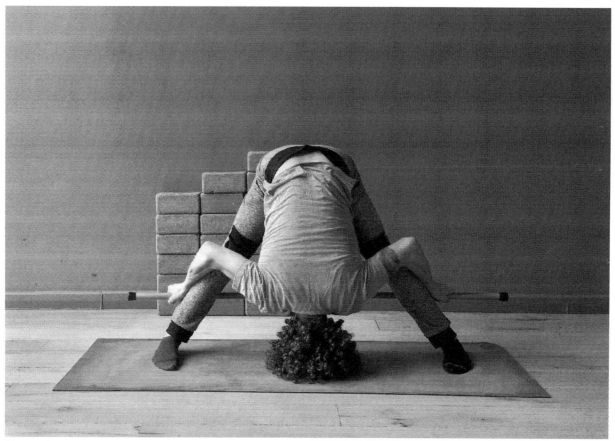

Rear view

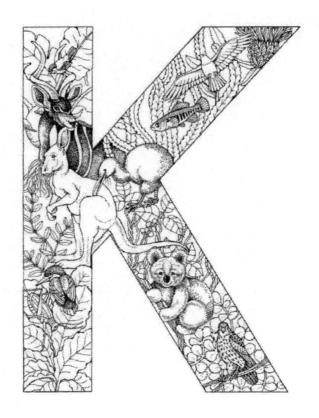

Kangaroo

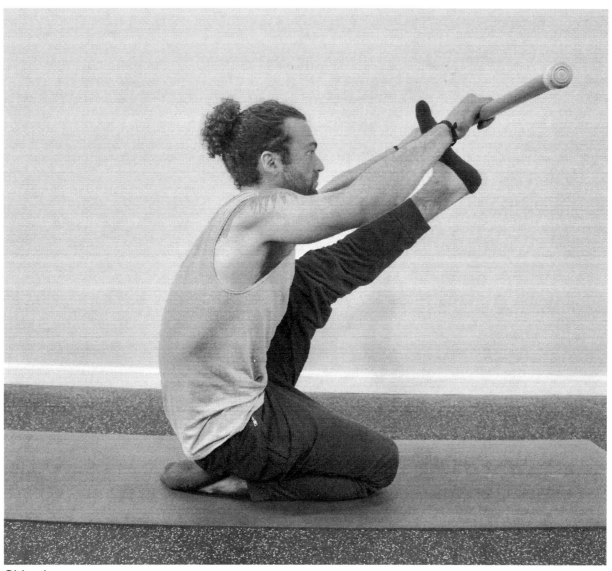

Side view

King Crab

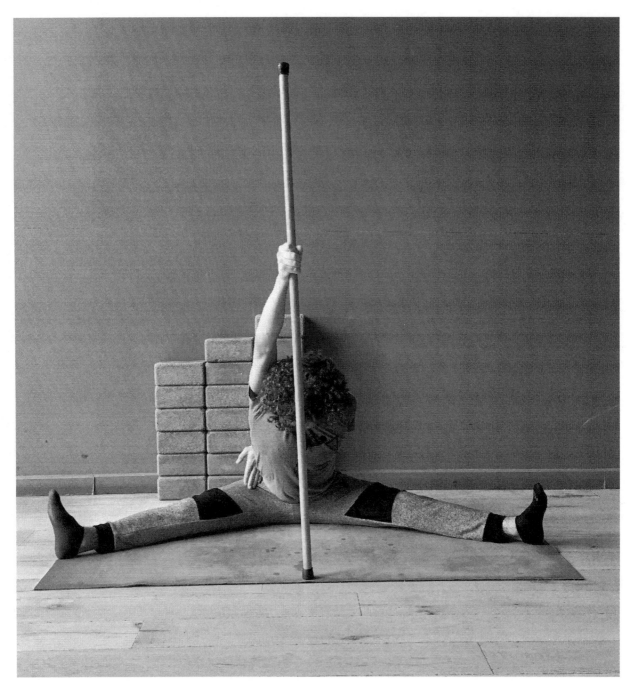

Front view

200

King P

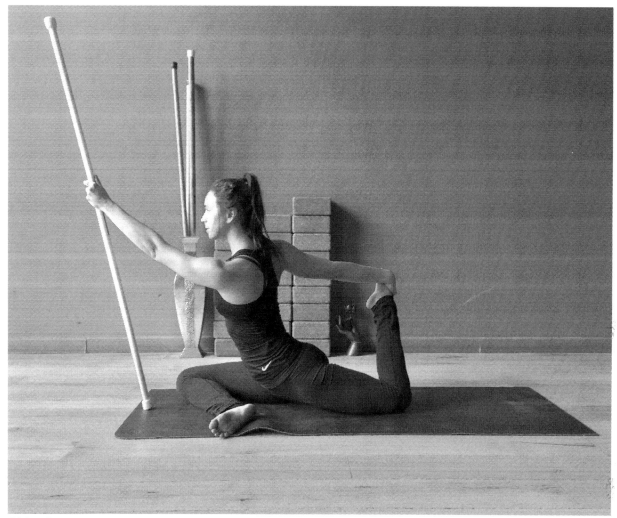
Side view

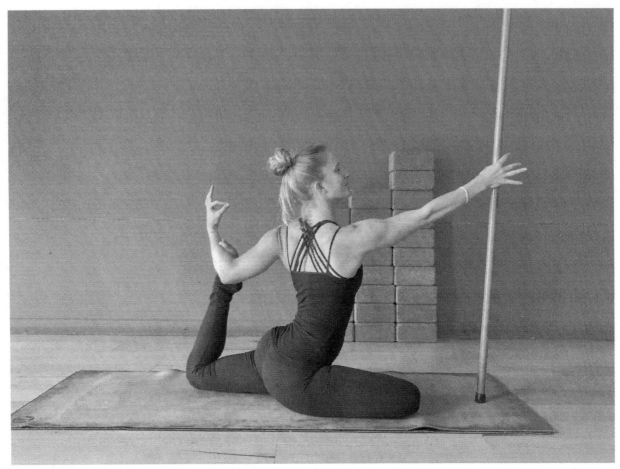

Side view

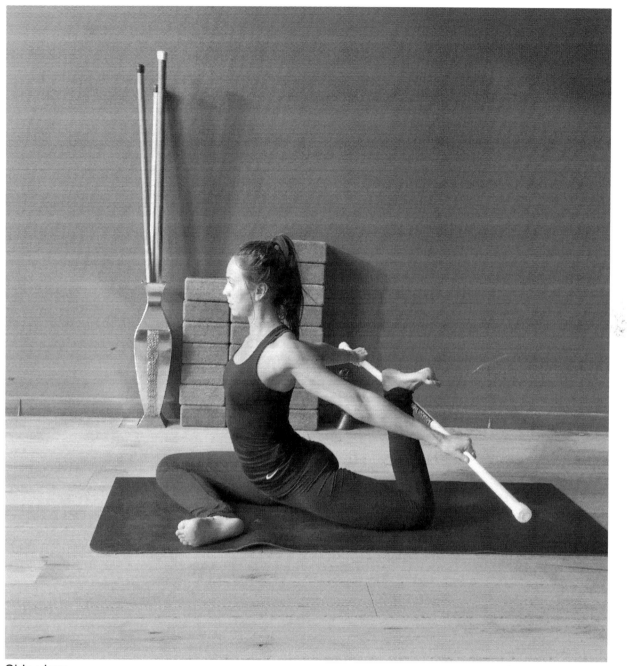

Side view

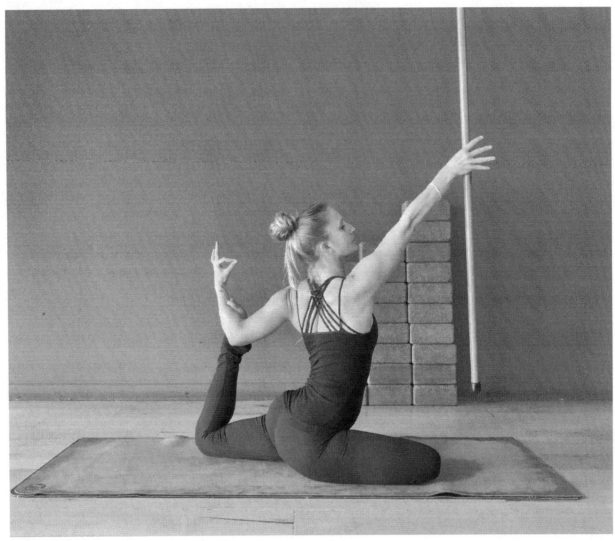

Front Side view

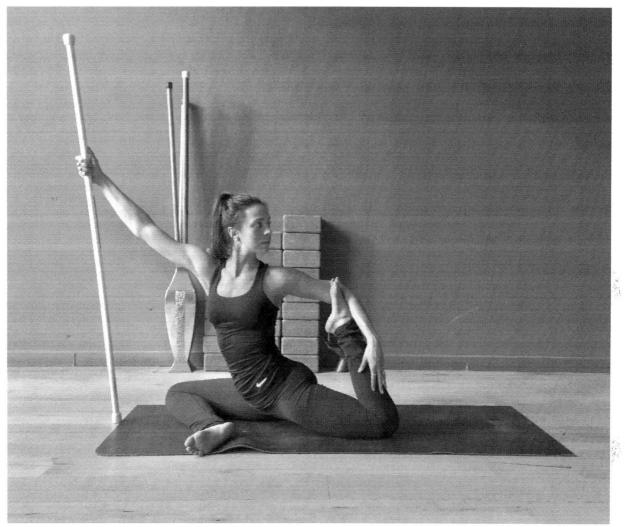

Front Side view

Kiss

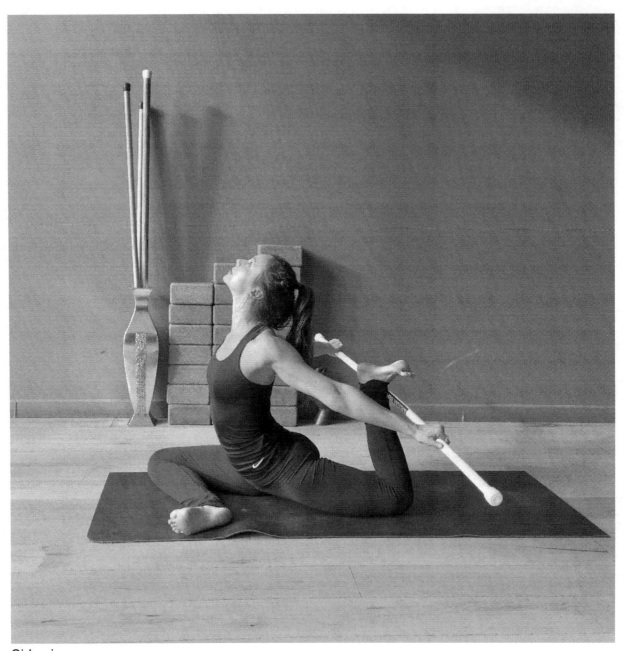

Side view

Komodo D

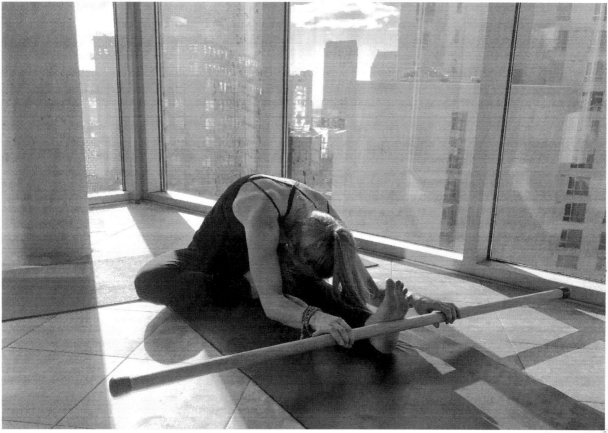

Front Side view

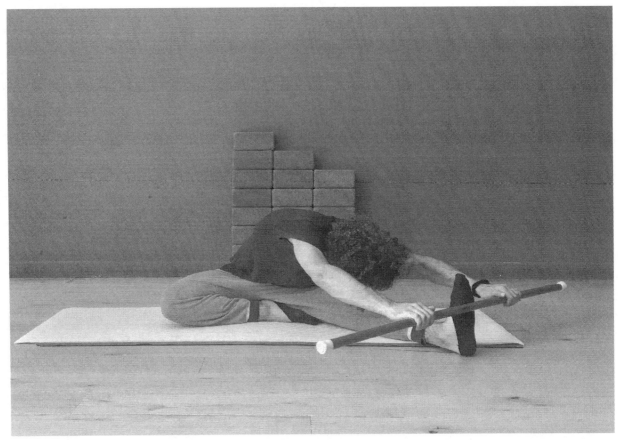

Front view

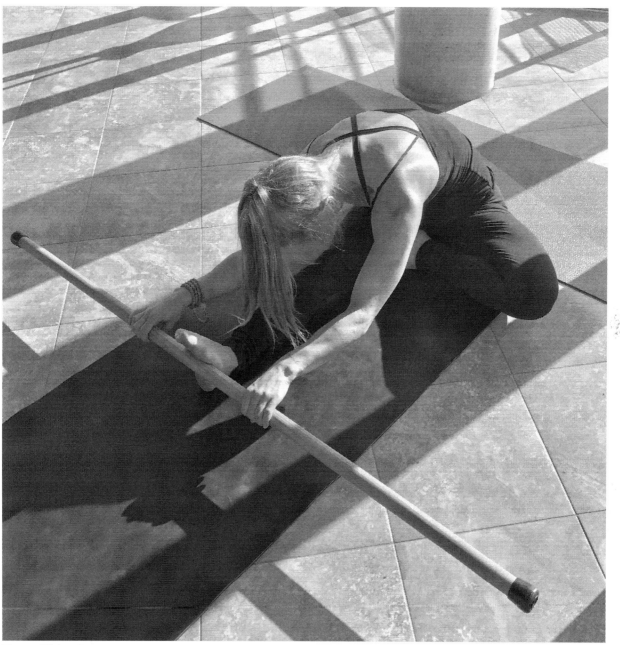

Front Side view

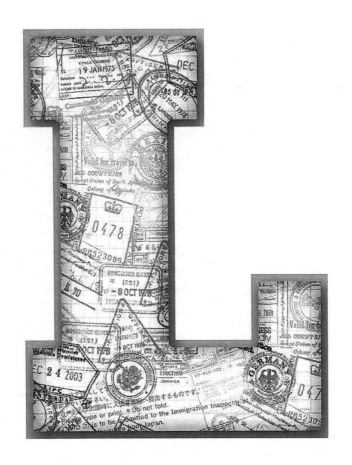

Ladybird

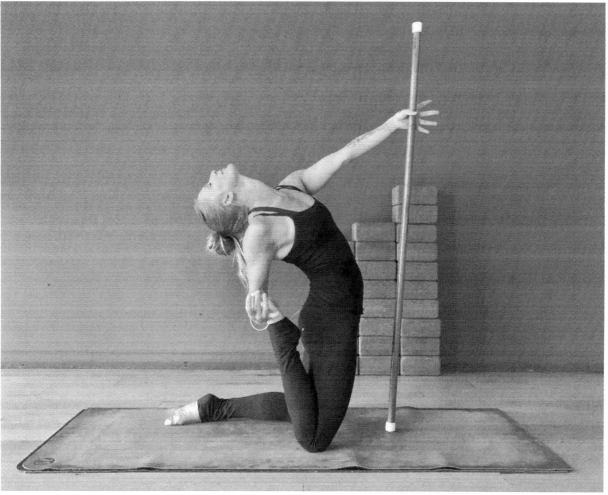

Side view

Lame Duck

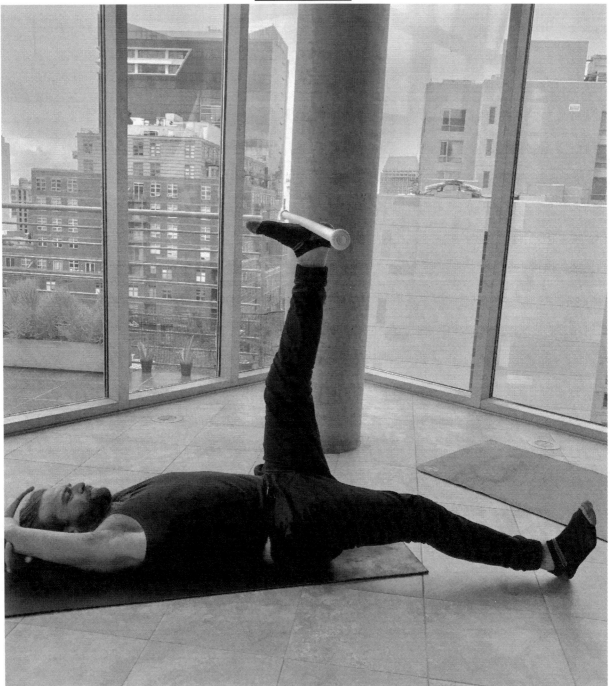

Side view

Libra

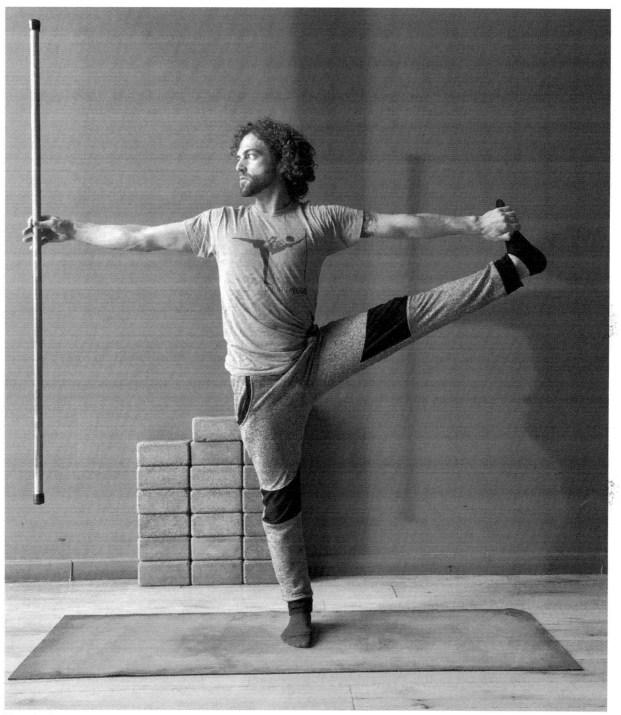
Front view

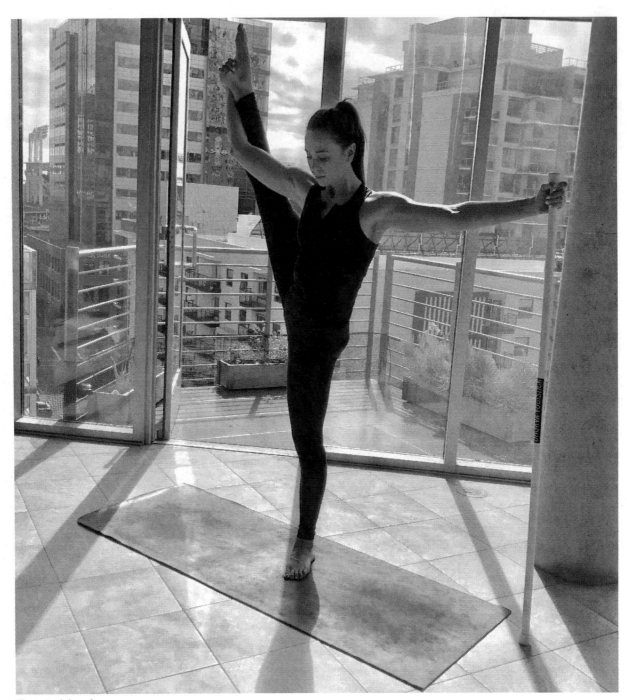

Front side view

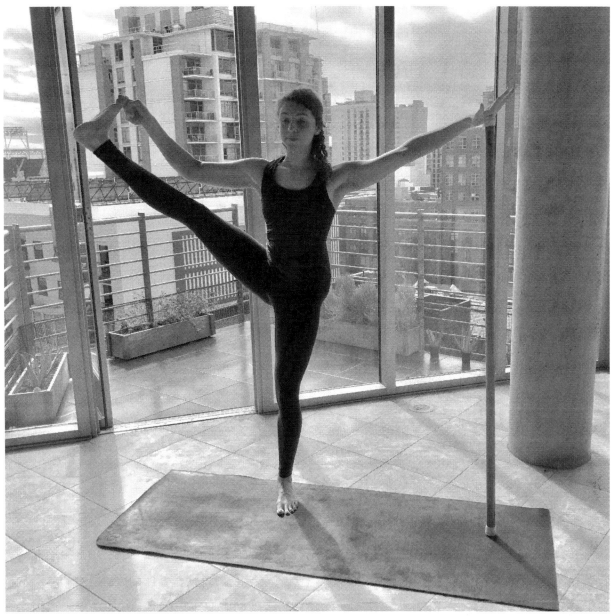

Front view

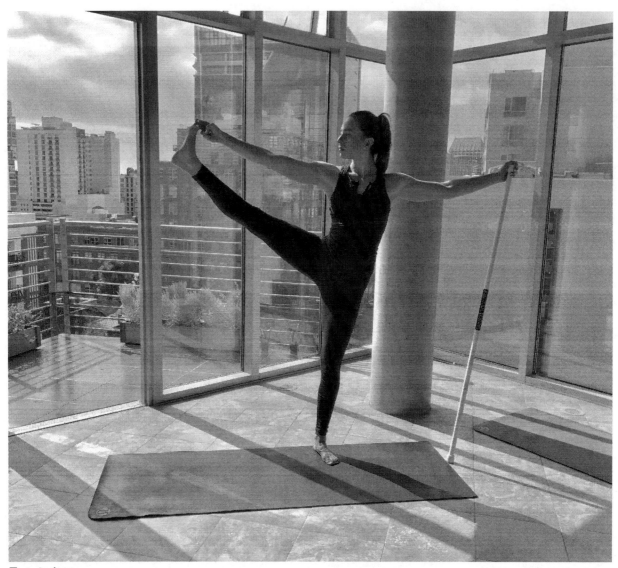

Front view

Limb

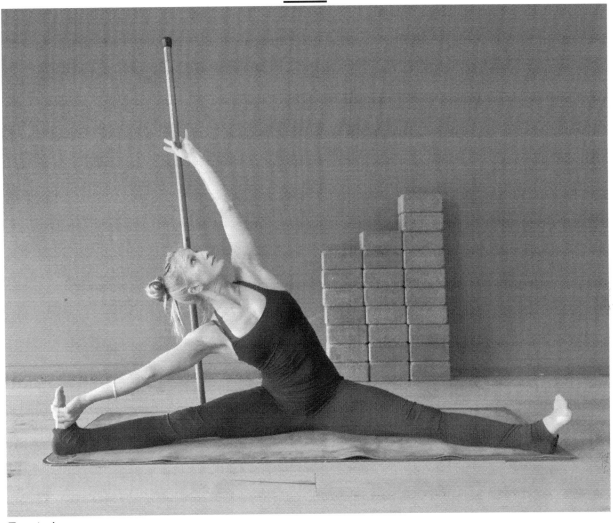

Front view

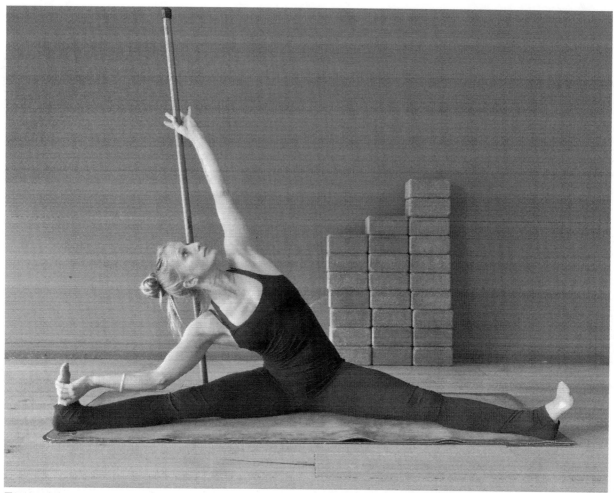
Front view

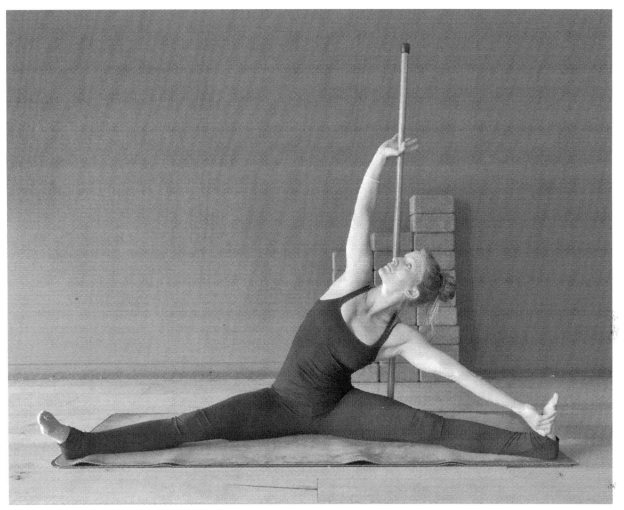

Front view

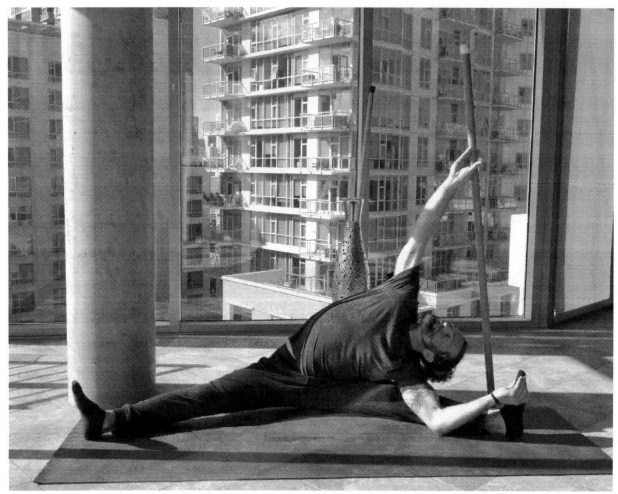

Front view

Llama

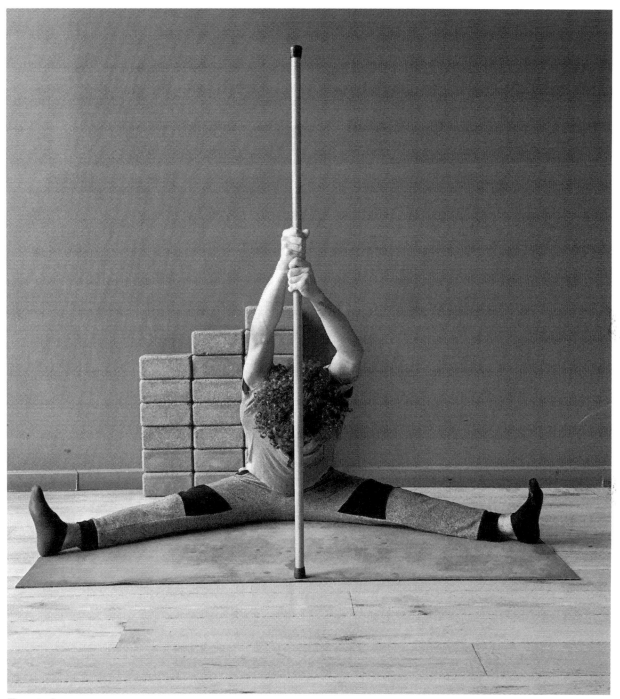
Front view

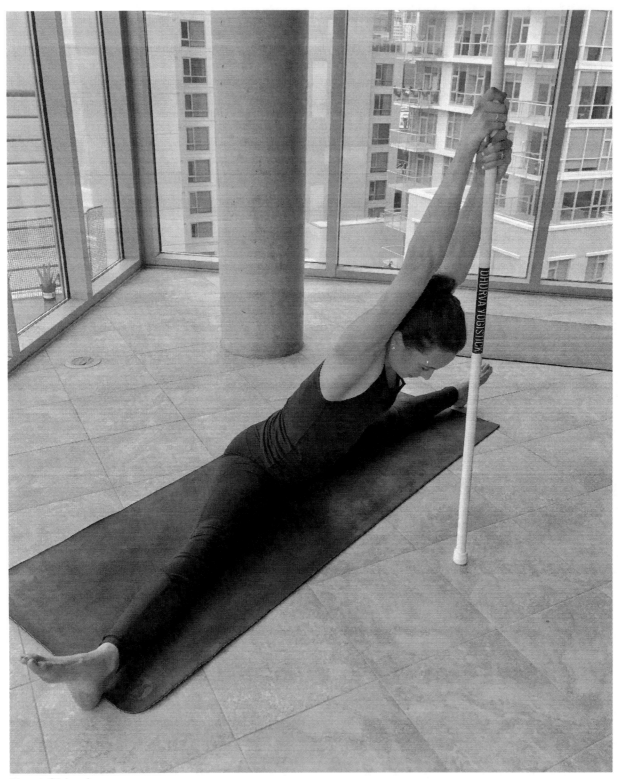

Front Side view

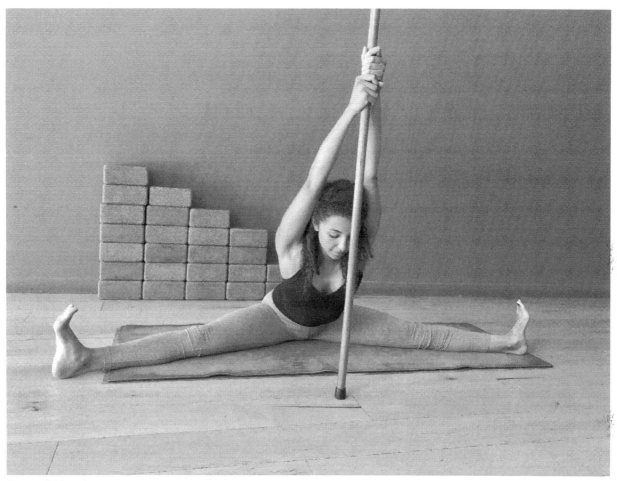
Front Side view

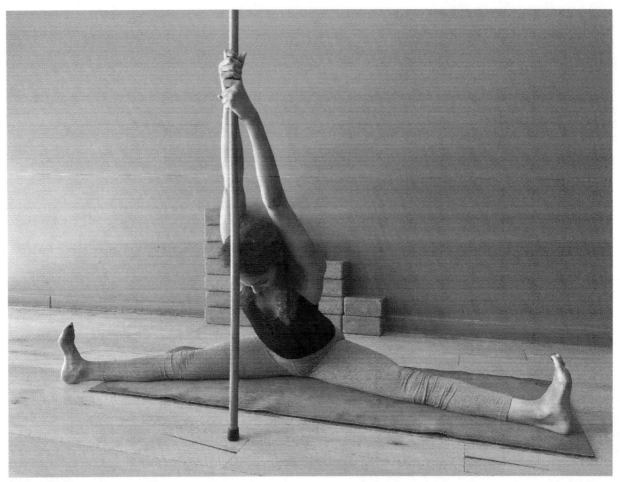

Front Side view

Love is Binding

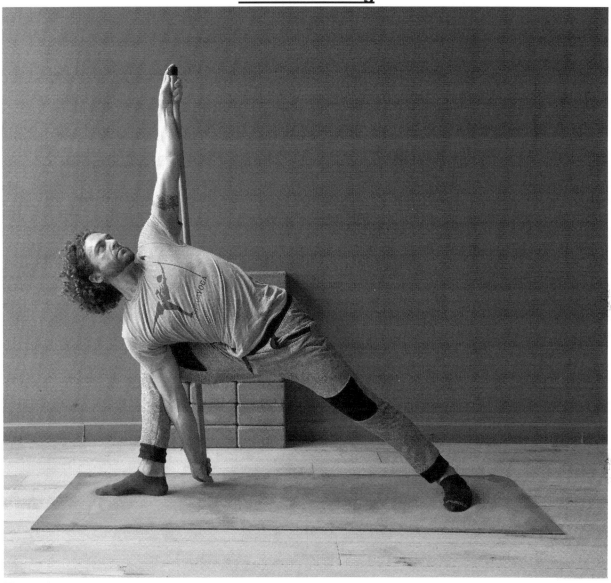

Front view

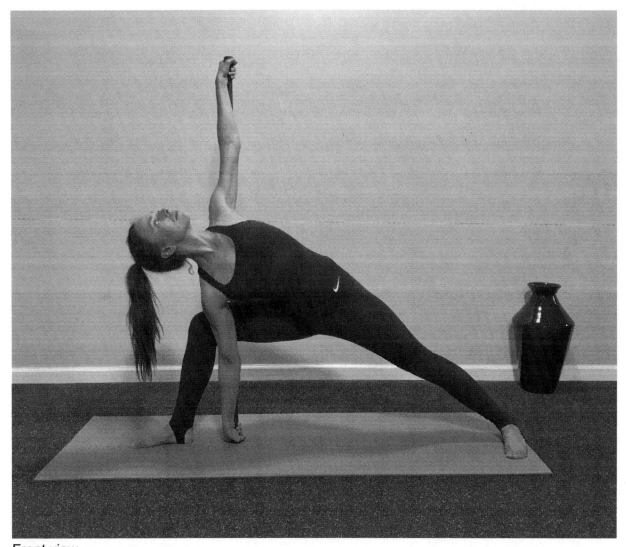

Front view

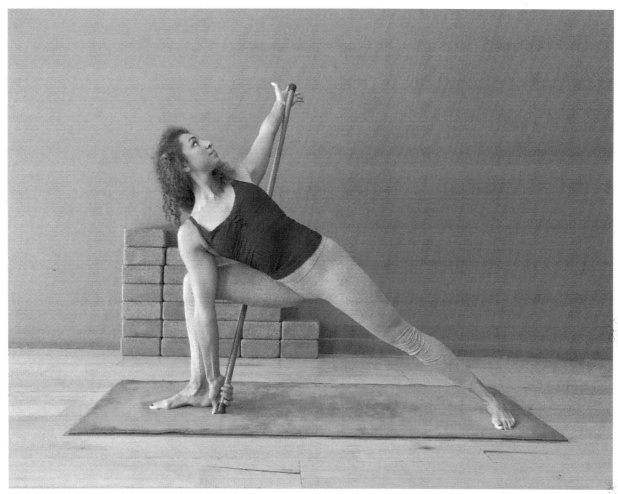

Front view

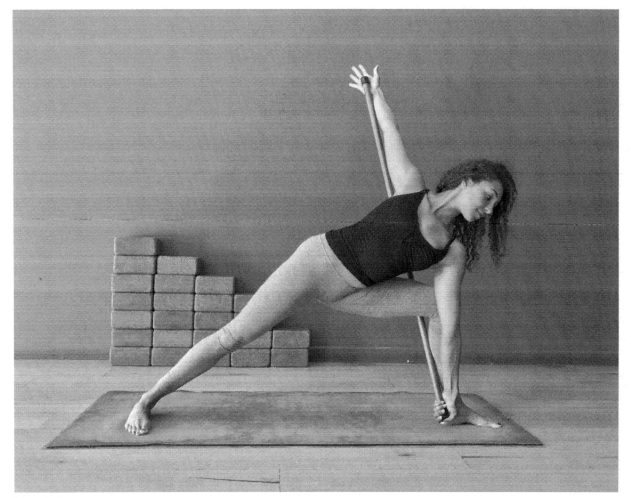

Front view

Loveseat

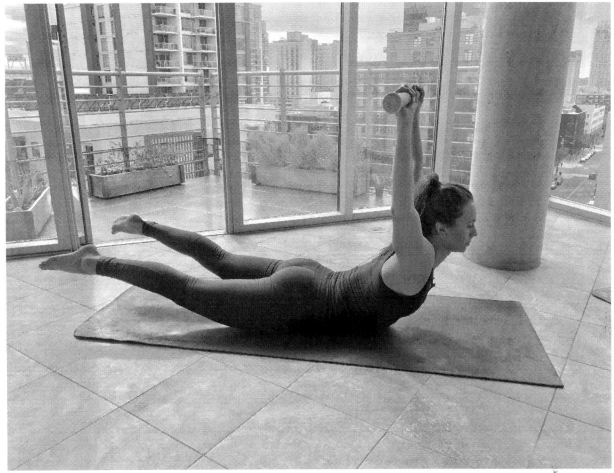
Side view

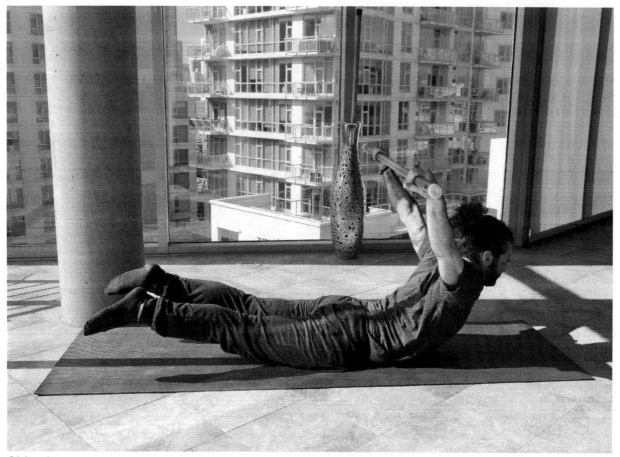

Side view

230

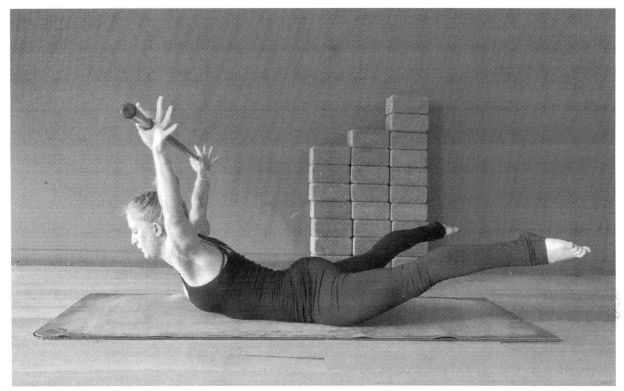

Side view

__Low Lunge__

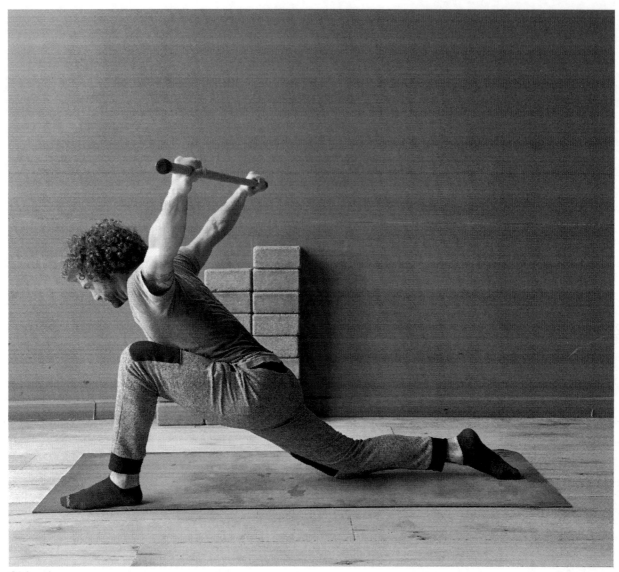
Side view

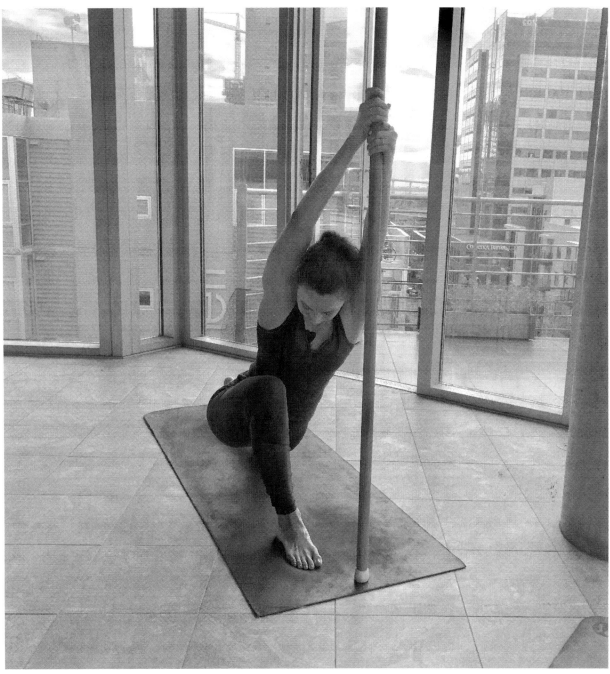

Front view

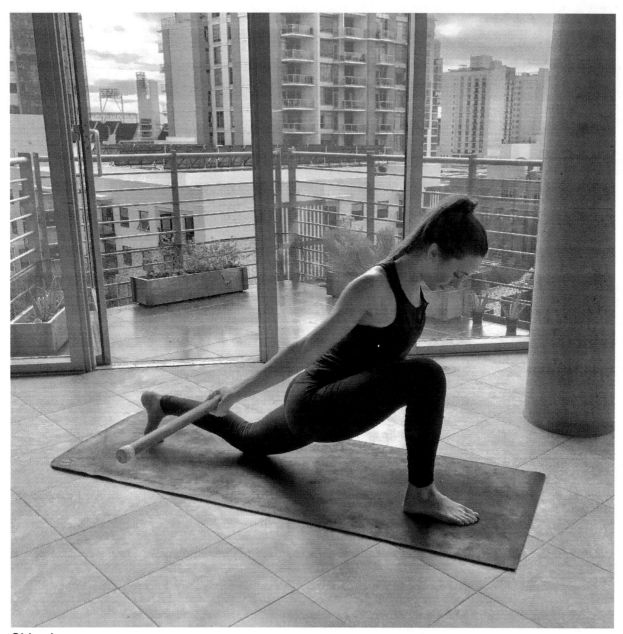

Side view

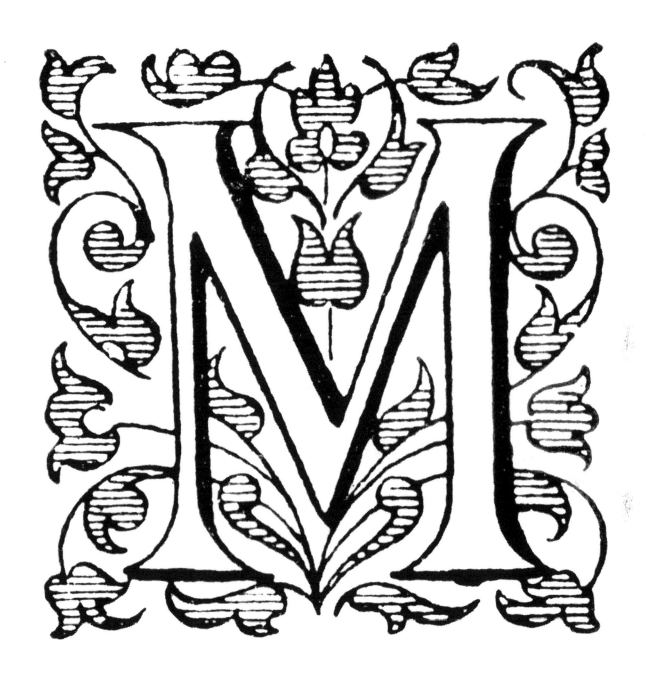

Magnetic Field

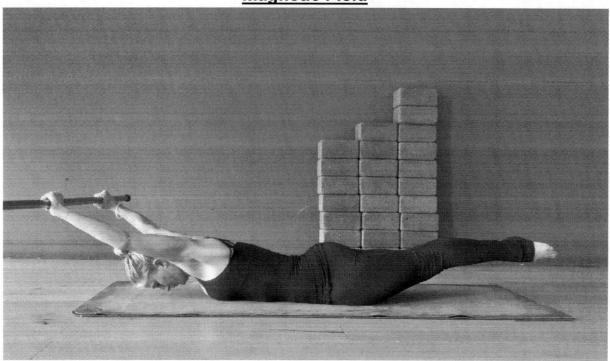

Side view

Magnetic Pole

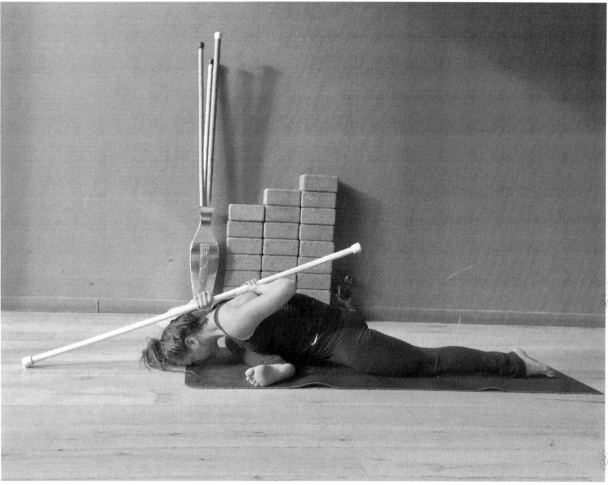

Side view

Meridian

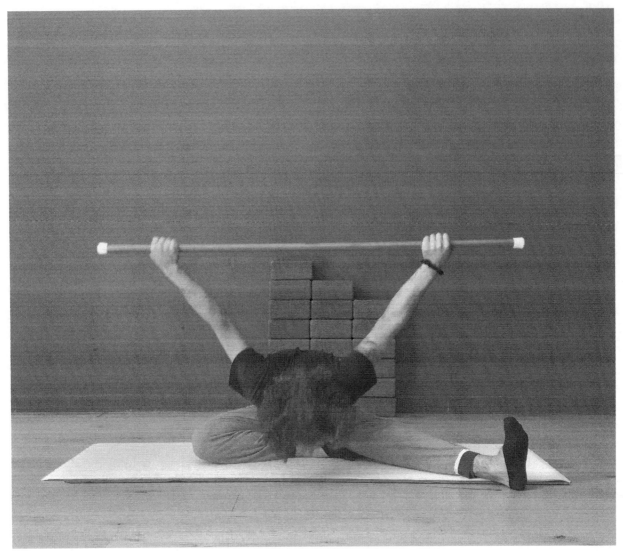
Front view

Meteor

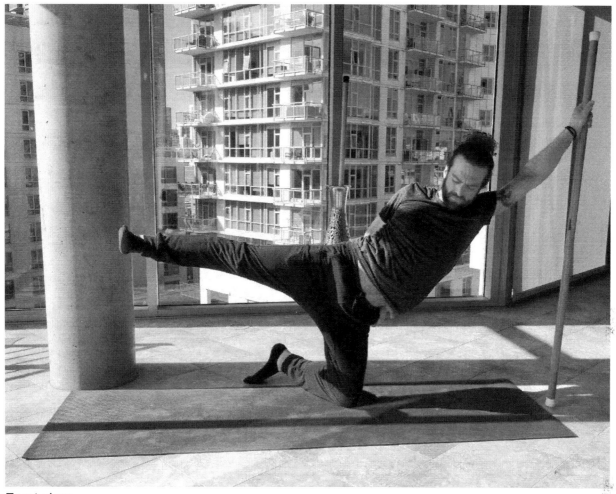

Front view

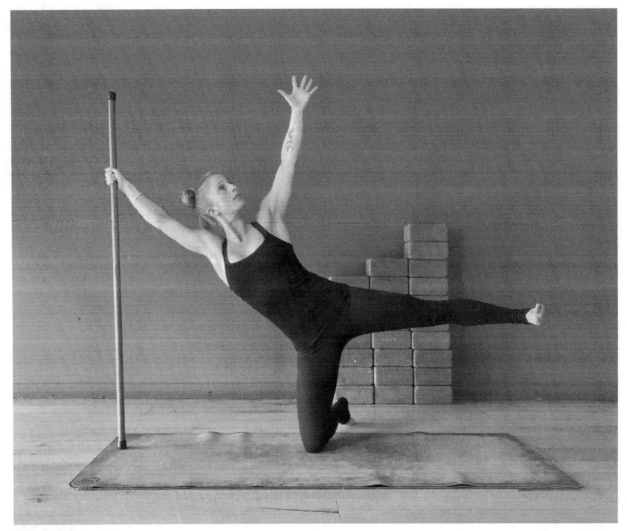

Front view

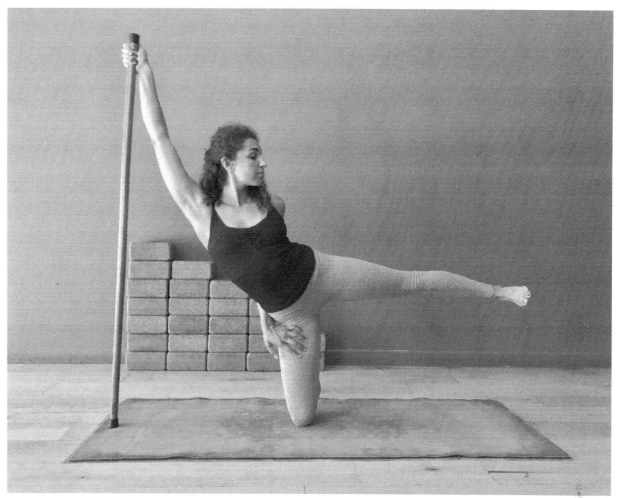

Front view

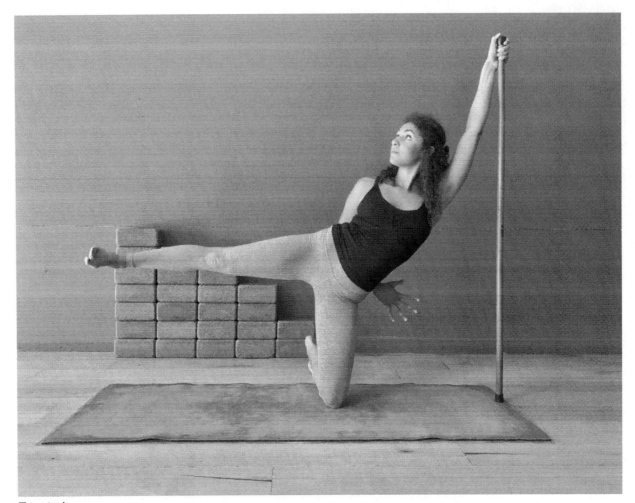

Front view

Miracle

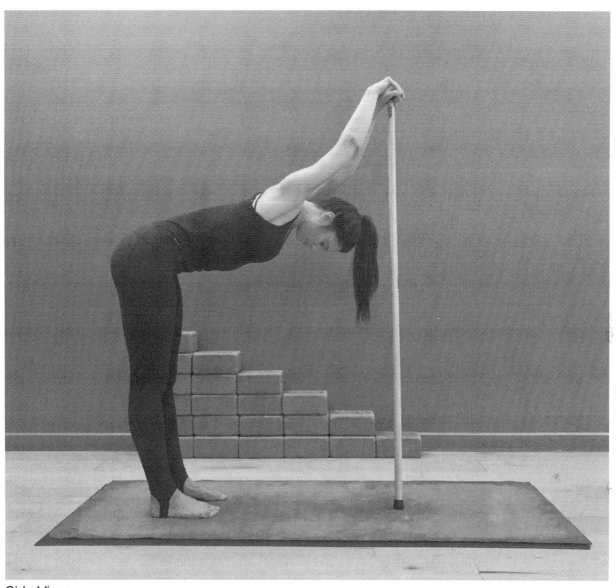

Side View

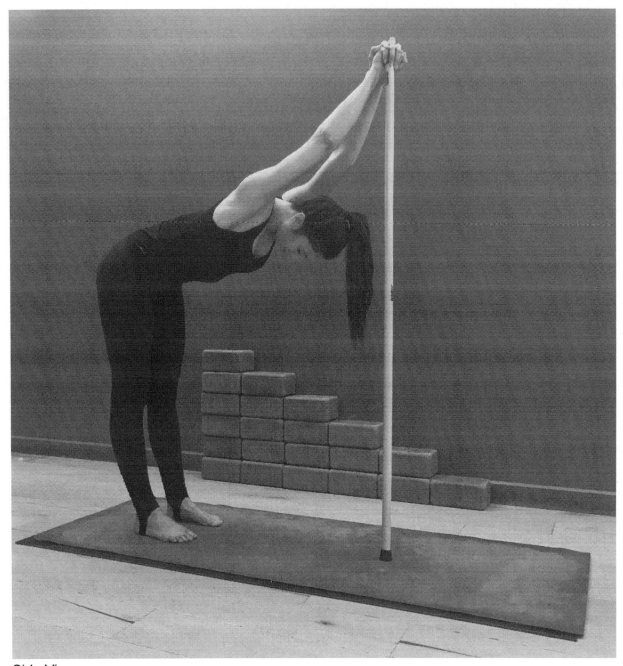

Side View

244

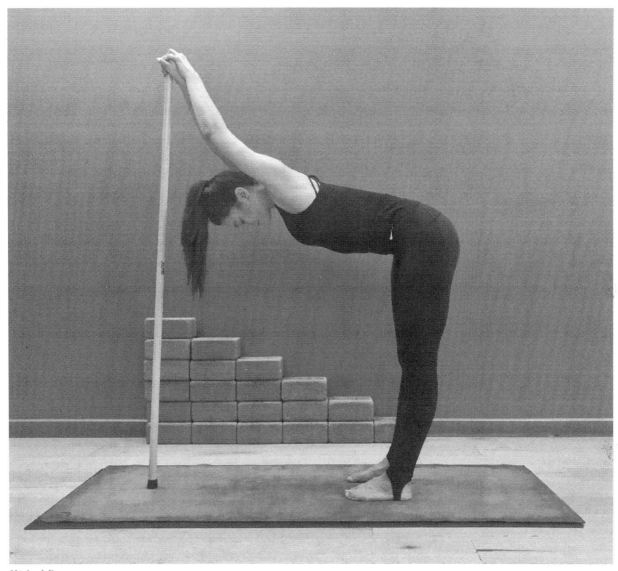

Side View

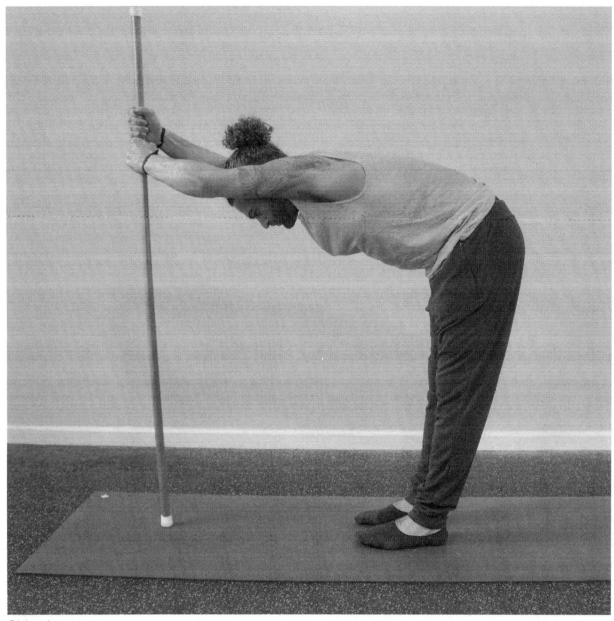
Side view

Miracle Belt

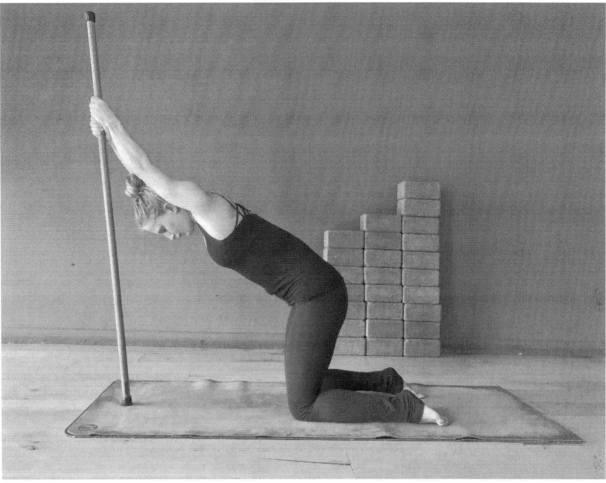

Side view

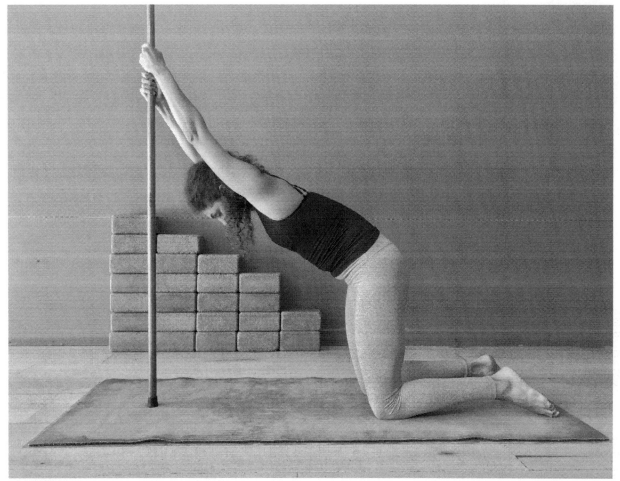

Side view

Monkey

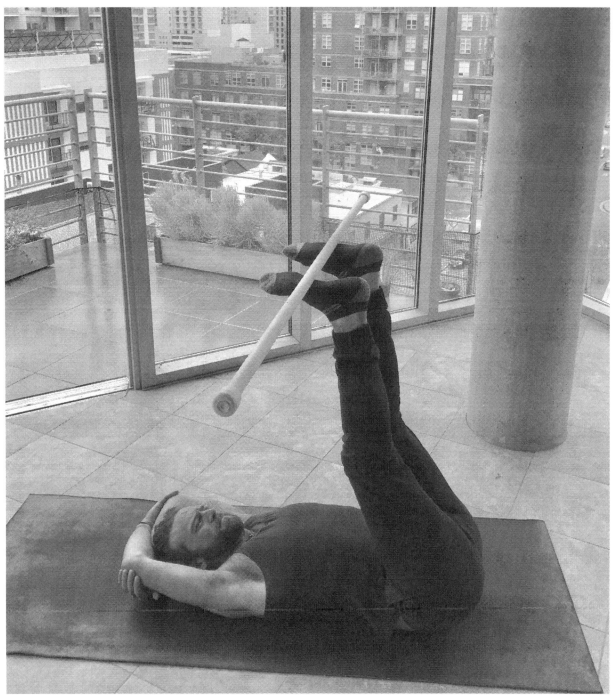

Front Side view

Mountain

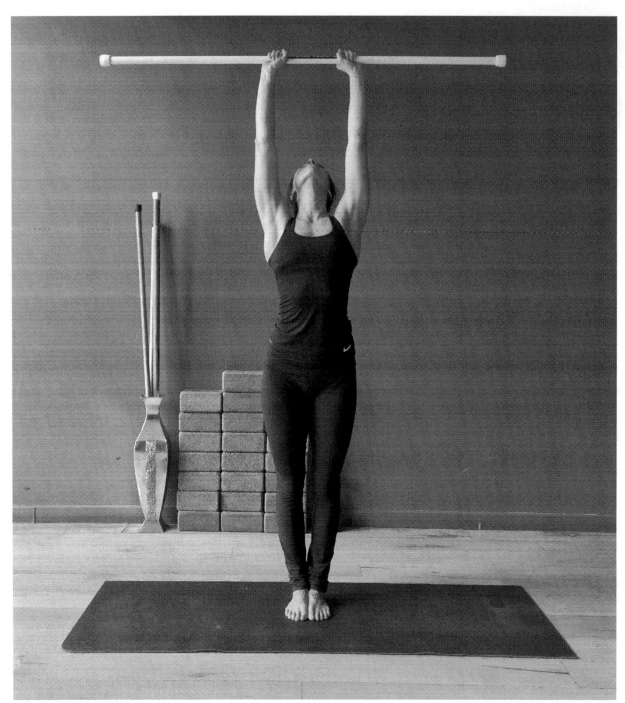

Front view

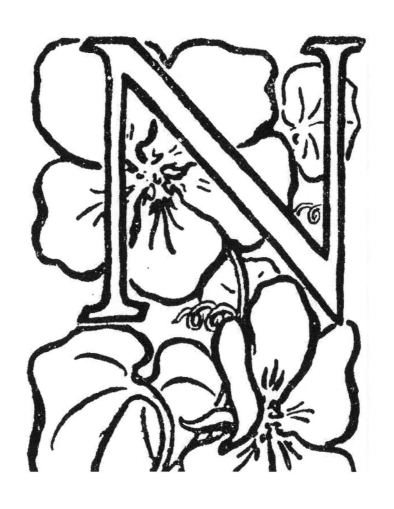

Namaste

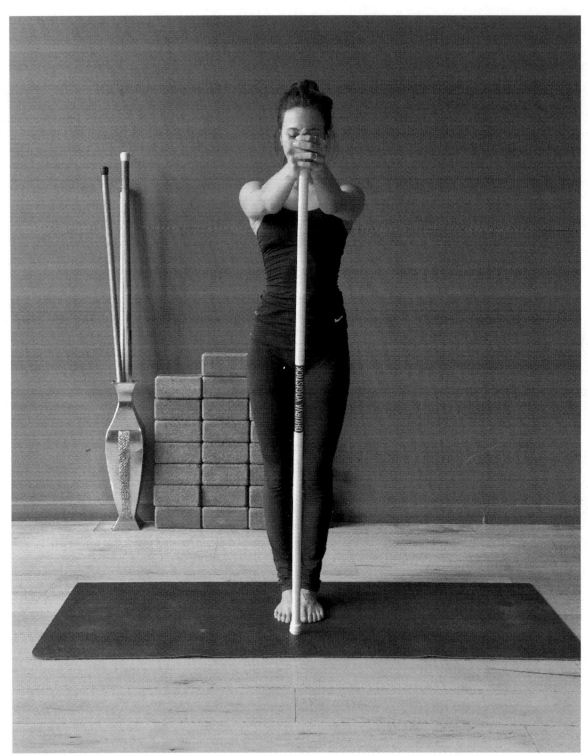

Front view

Nature

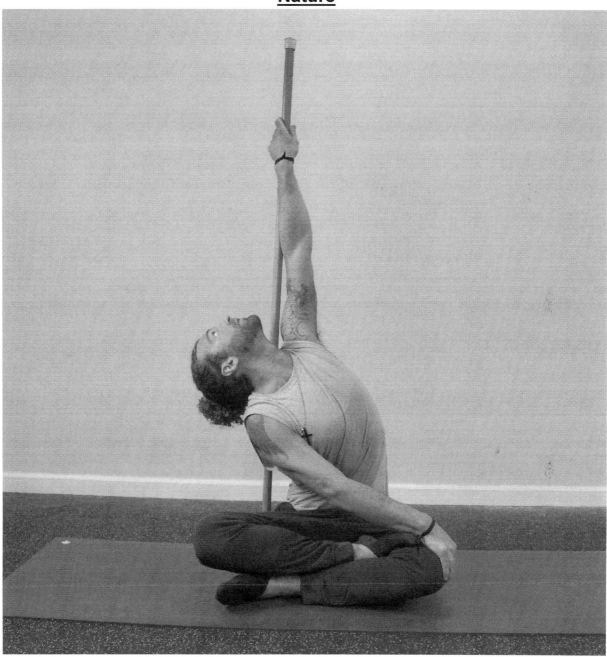

Front view

Noah's Ark

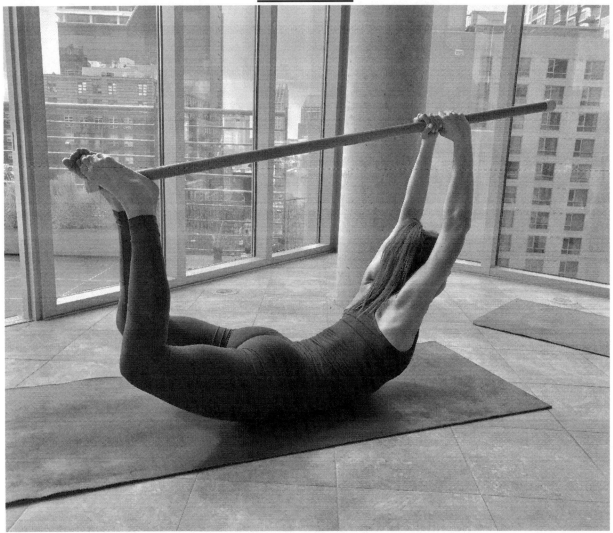

Side view

Non Resistance

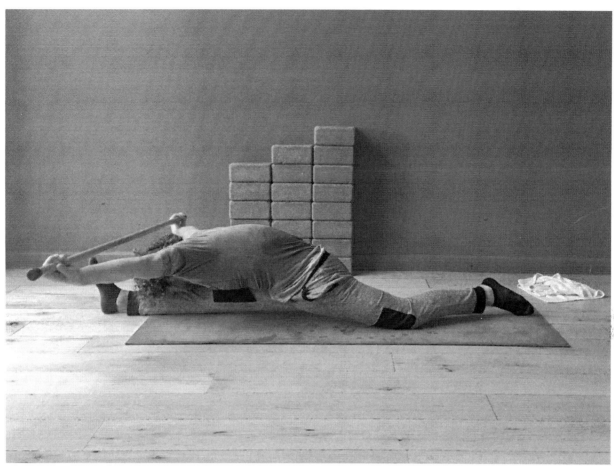
Side view

Not So Easy

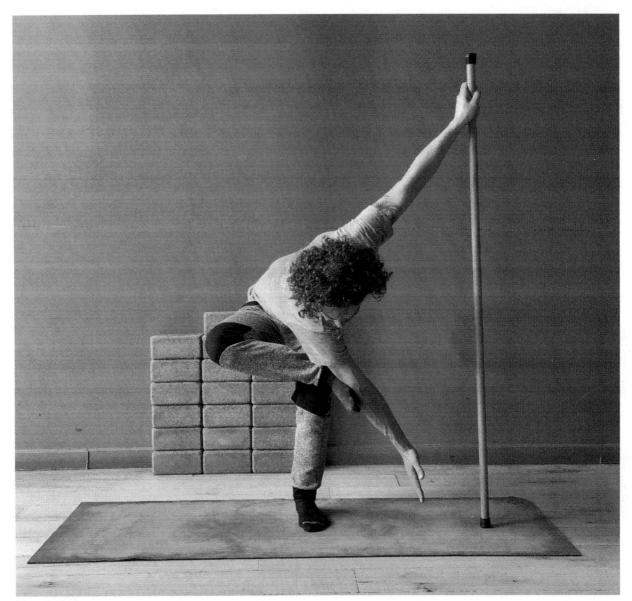

Front view

Nova

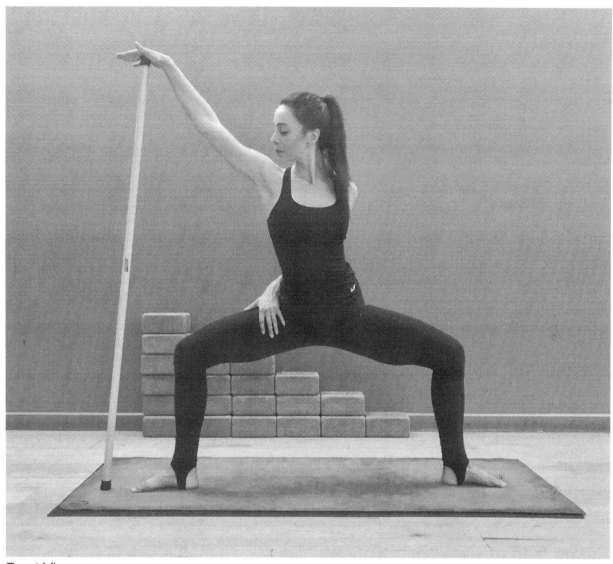

Front View

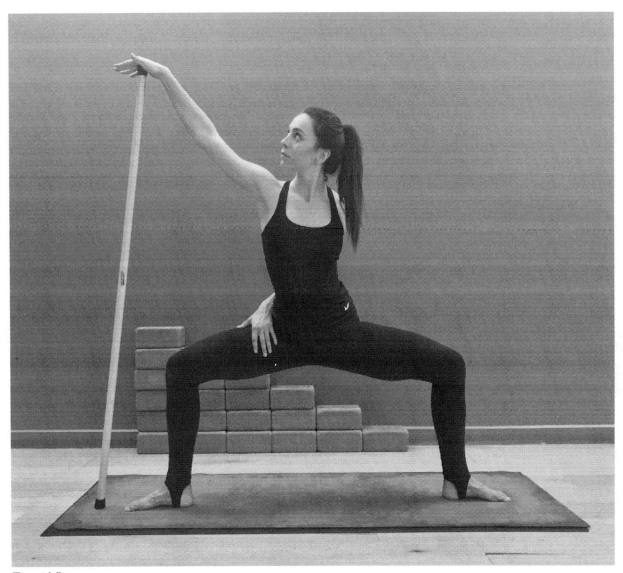

Front View

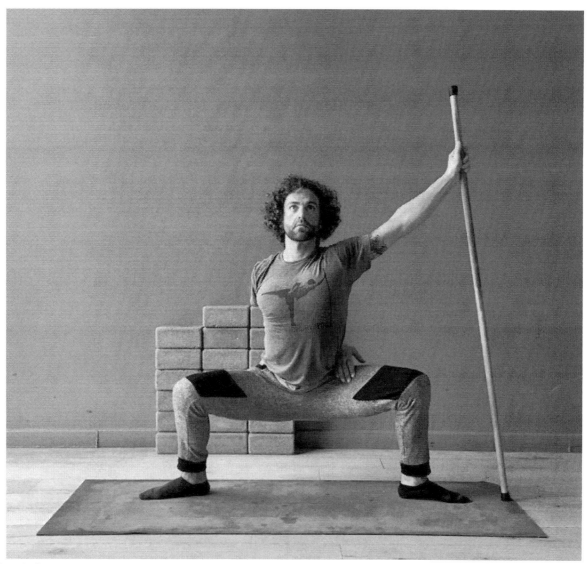

Front view

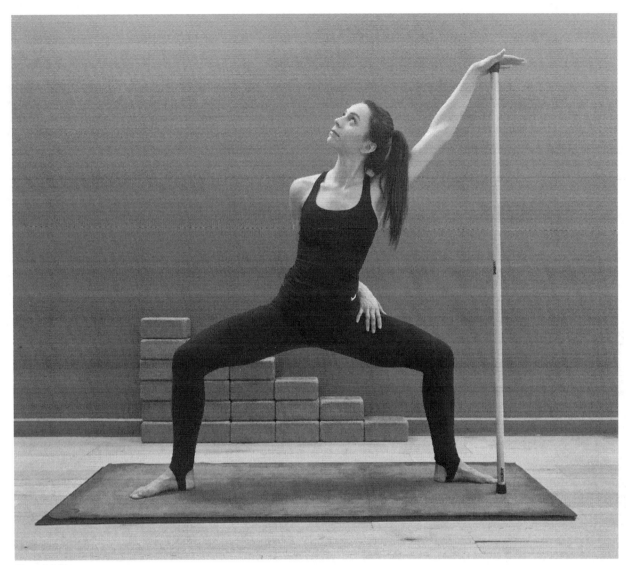
Front View

Number 4

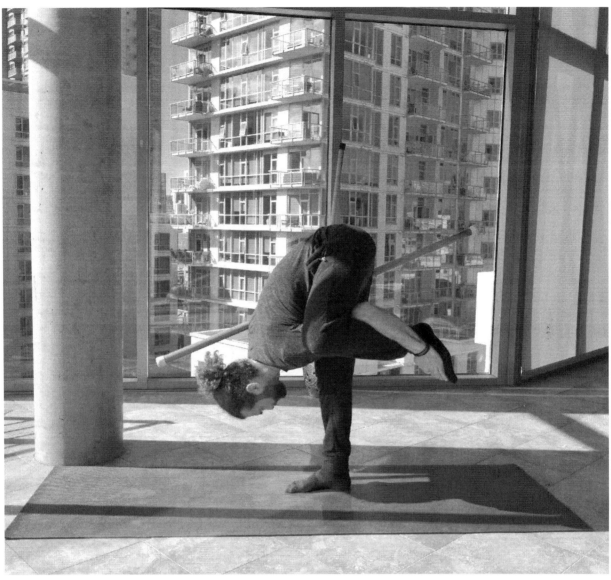

Side view

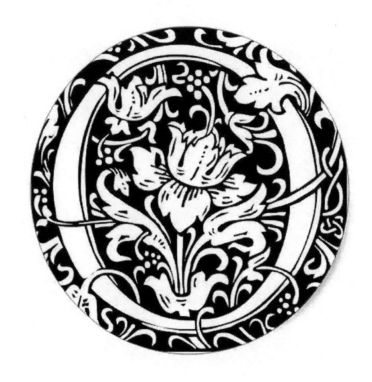

Olympic

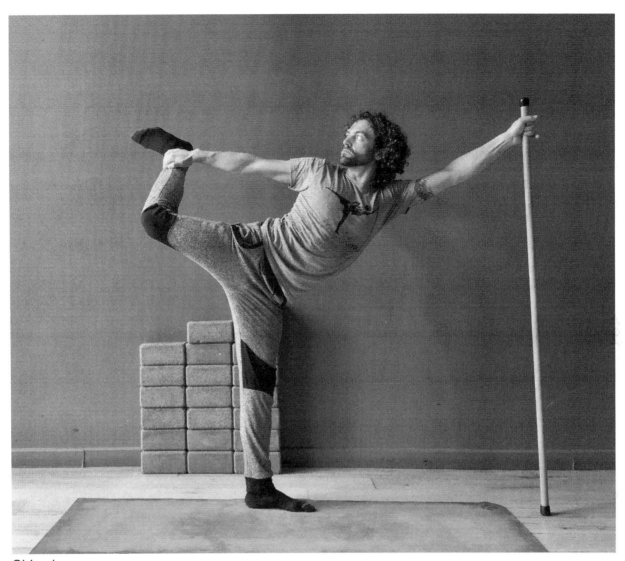

Side view

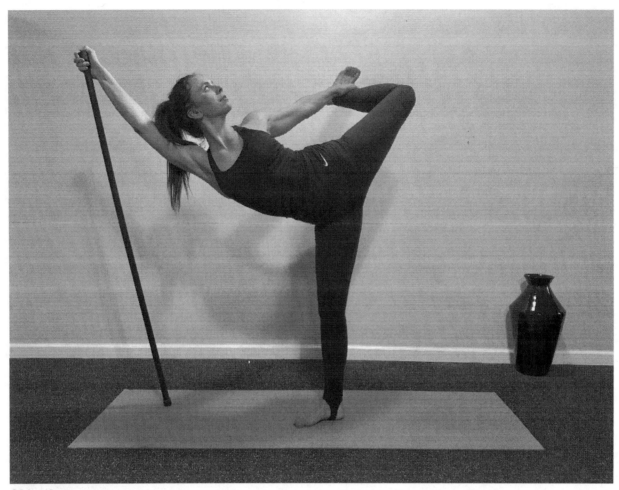

Side view

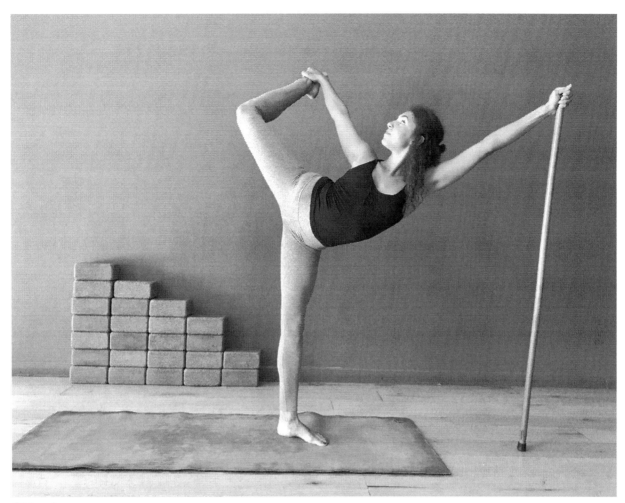

Side view

Open Cluster

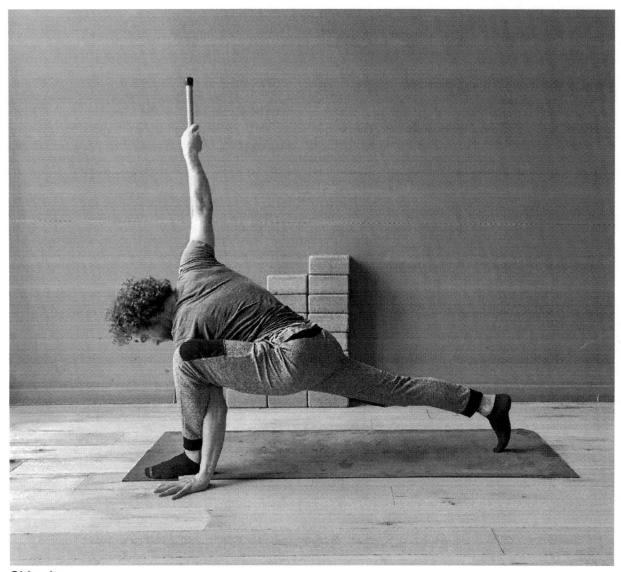

Side view

Open Heart

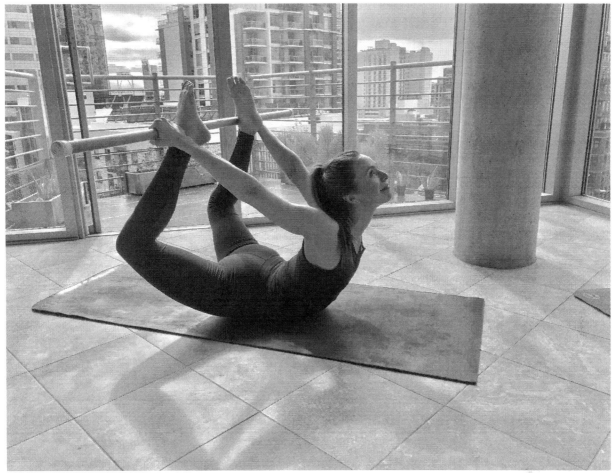

Side view

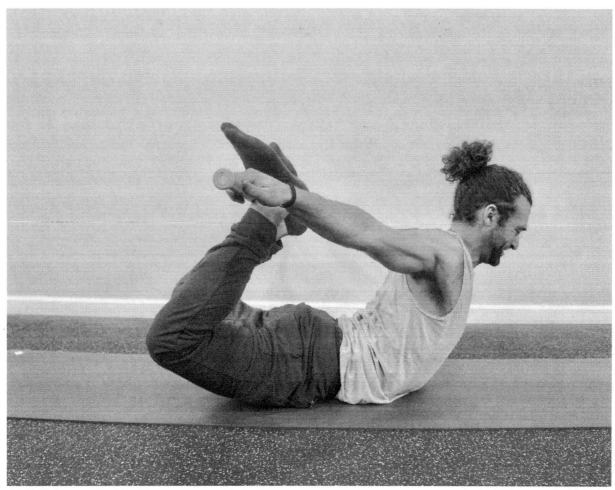
Side view

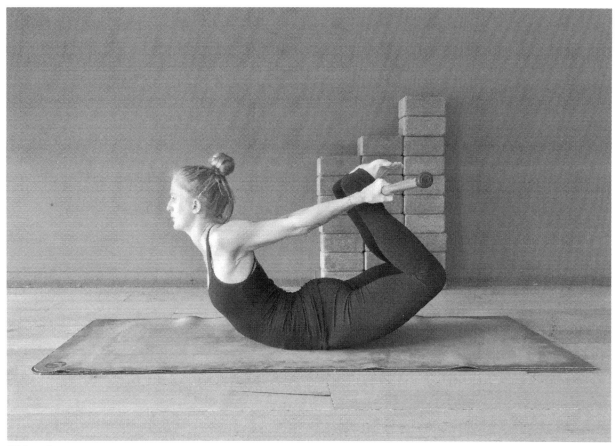

Side view

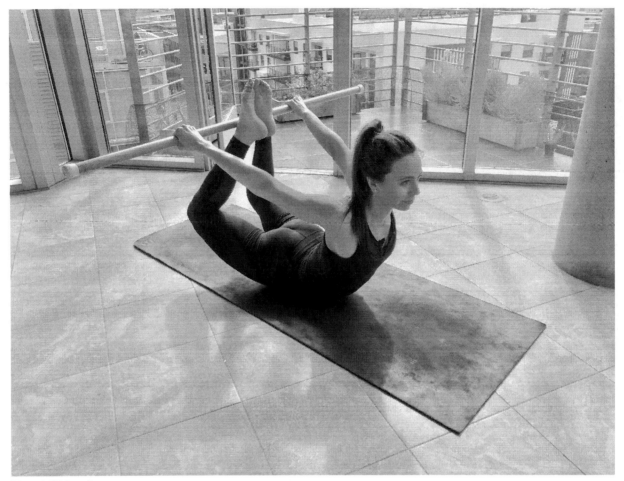

Front Side view

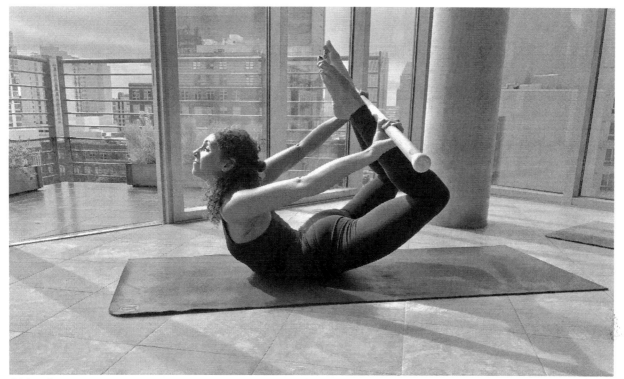
Side view

271

Opposition

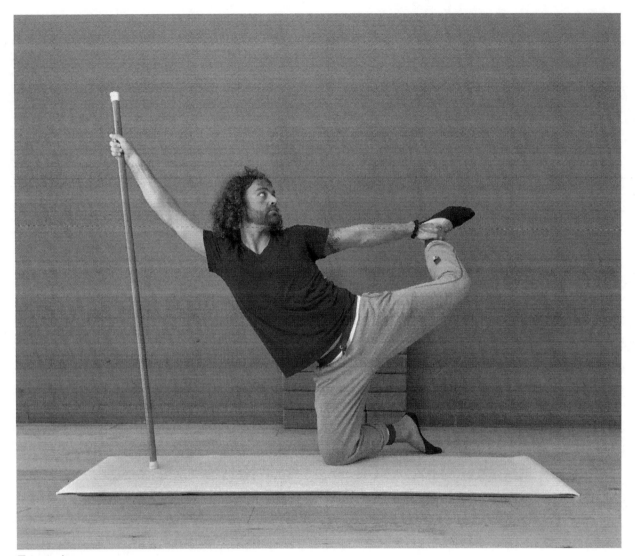

Front view

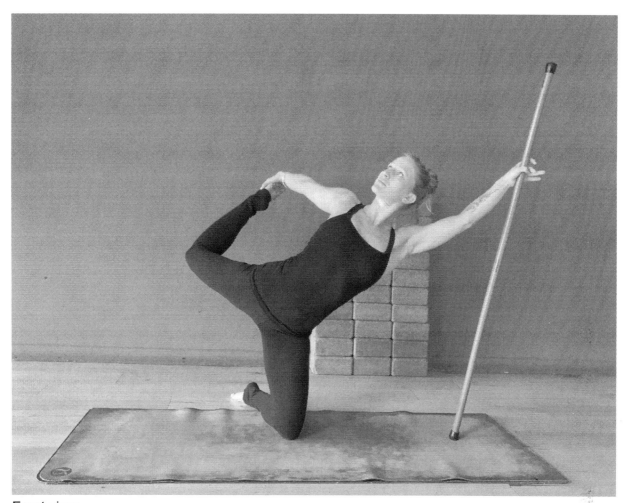

Front view

Orchid

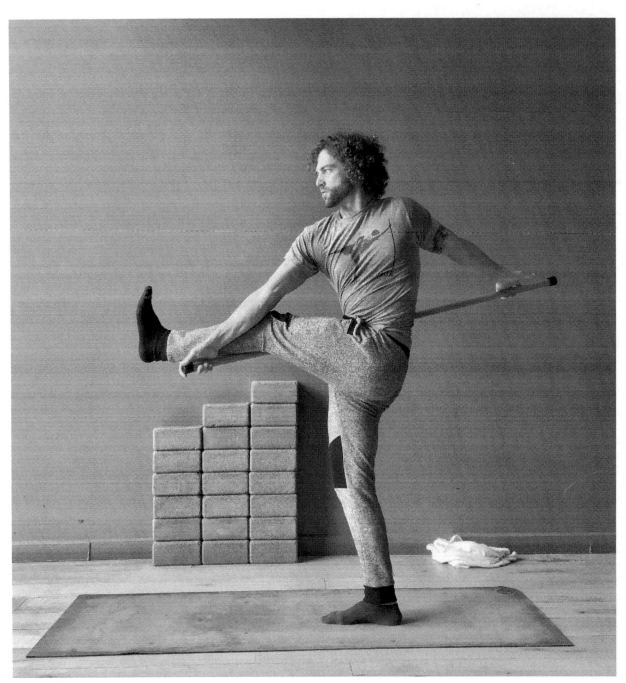
Side view

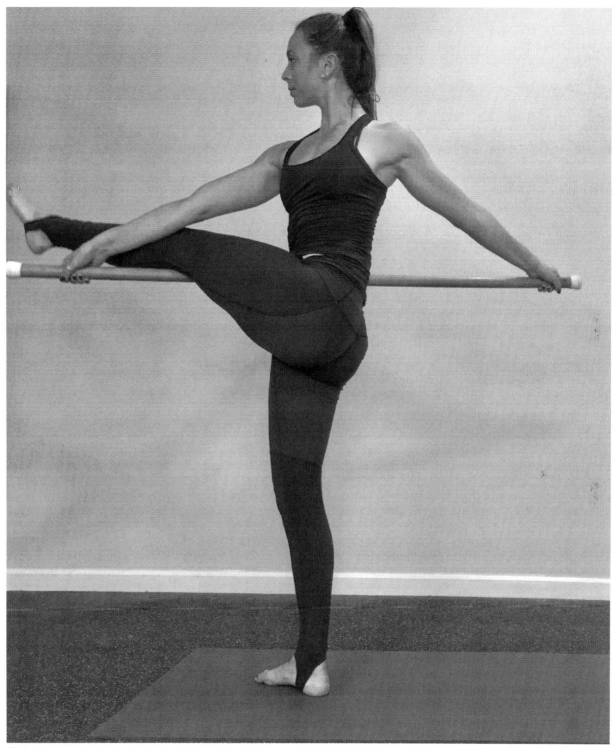
Side view

Ostriche

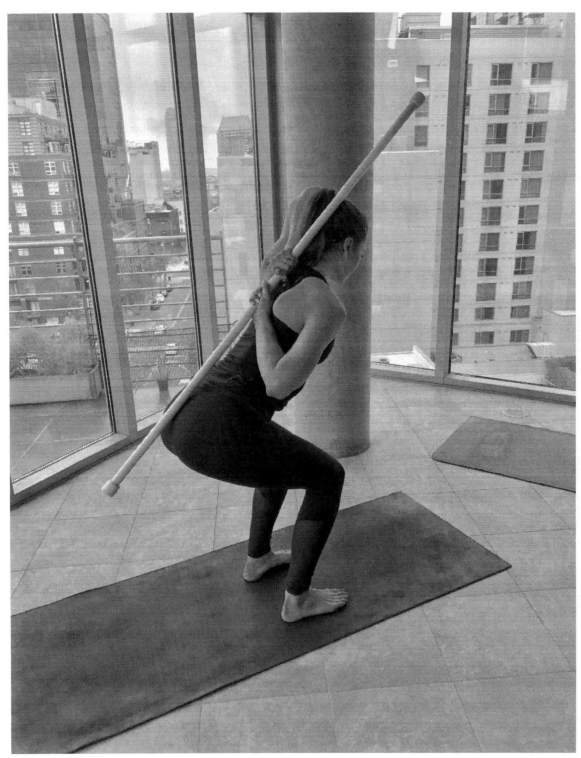

Rear Side View
276

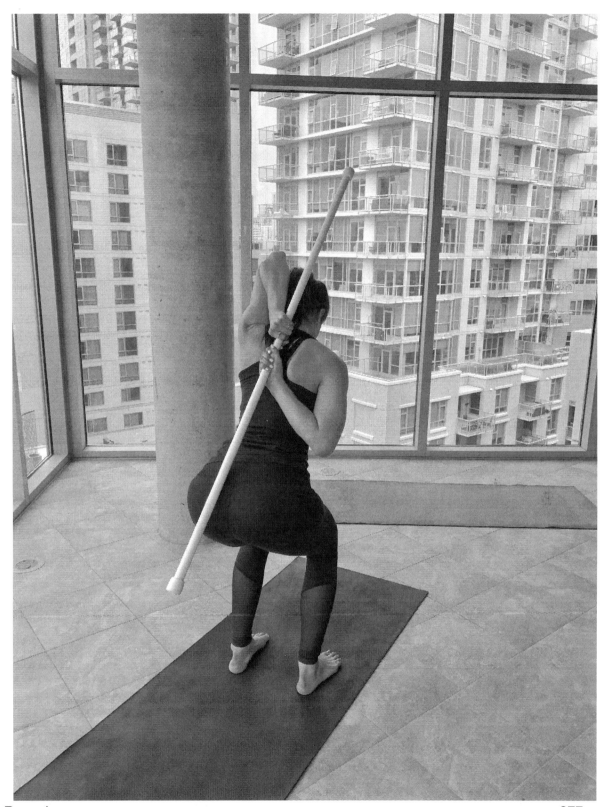

Rear view

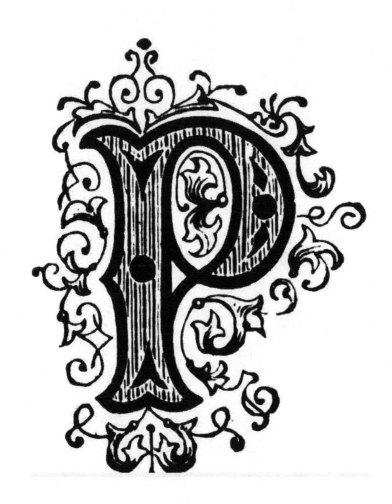

278

Patience

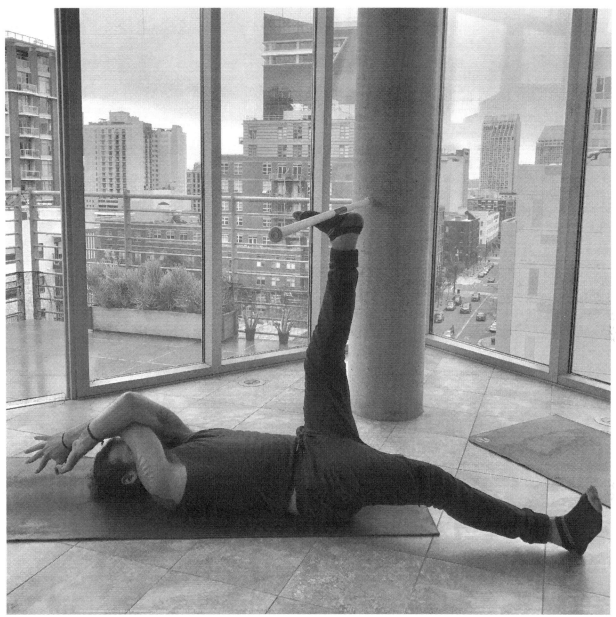

Side view

Pigeon

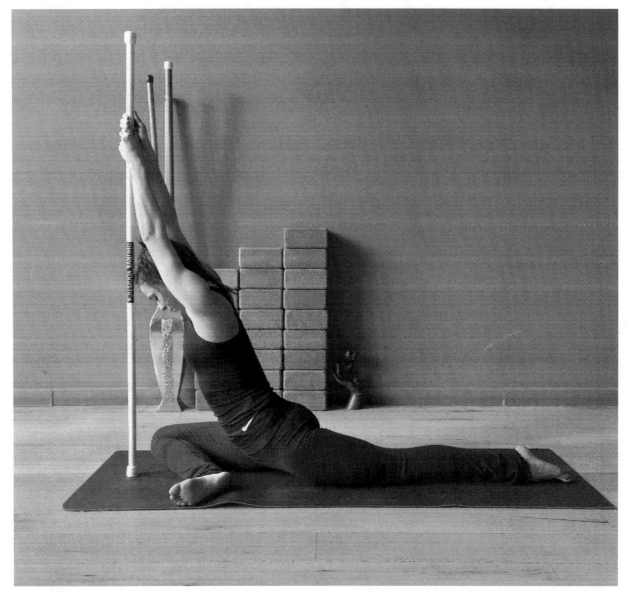

Side view

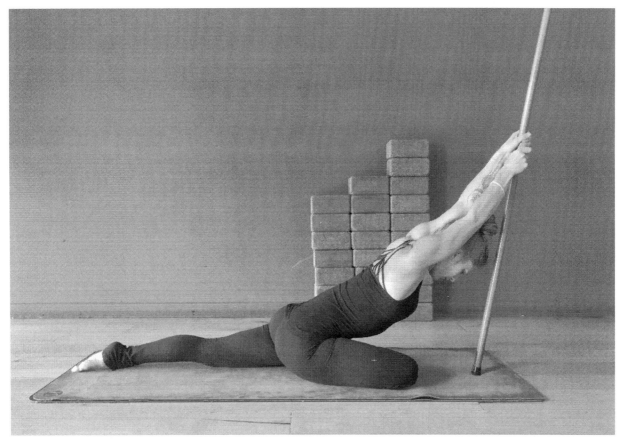
Side view

Pistol

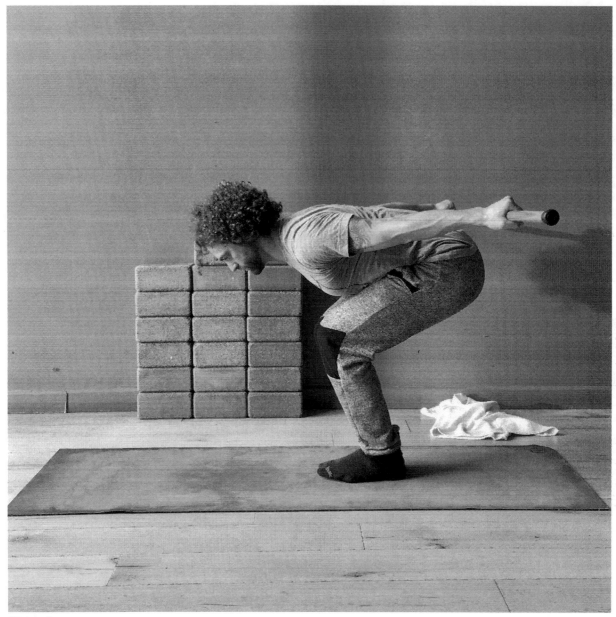
Side view

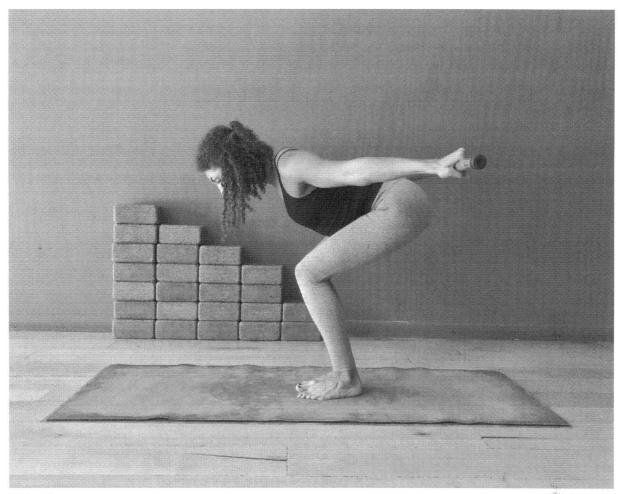
Side view

Plow

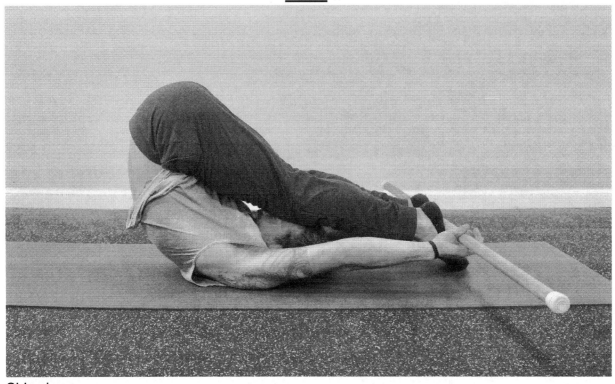

Side view

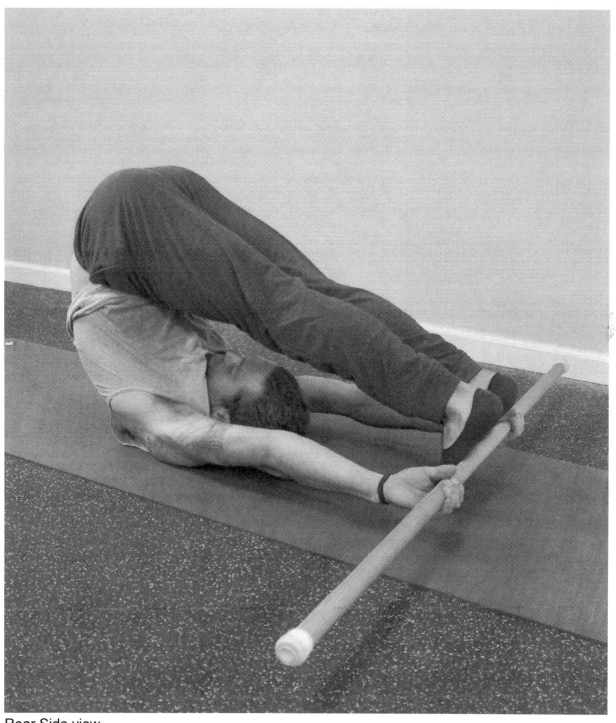

Rear Side view

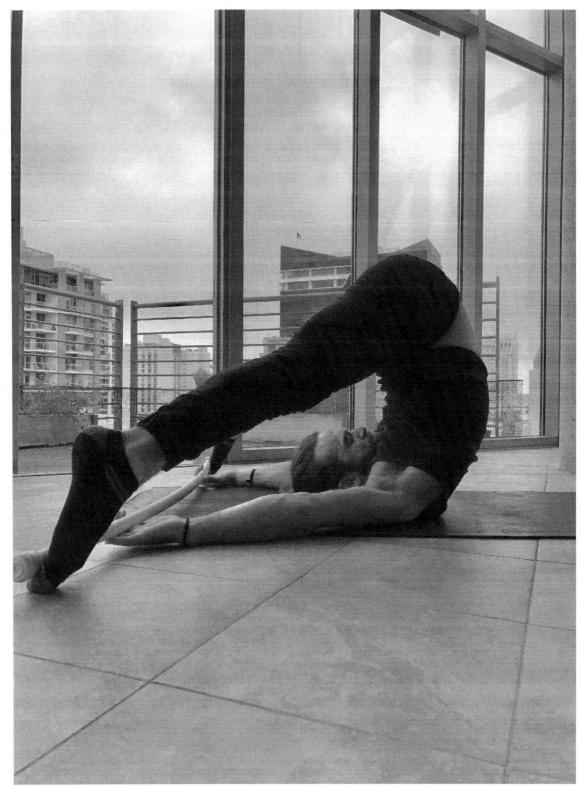

Side view
286

Porcupine

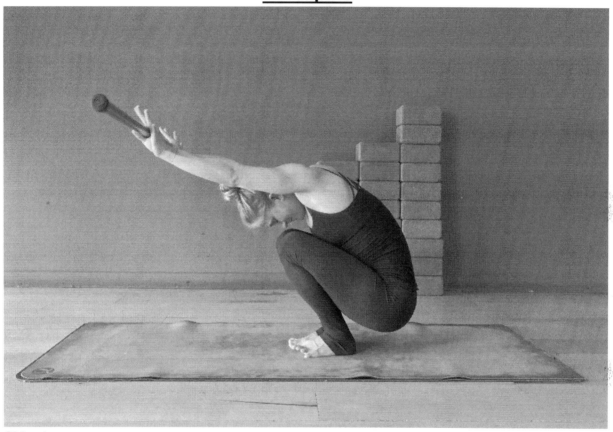

Side view

Power

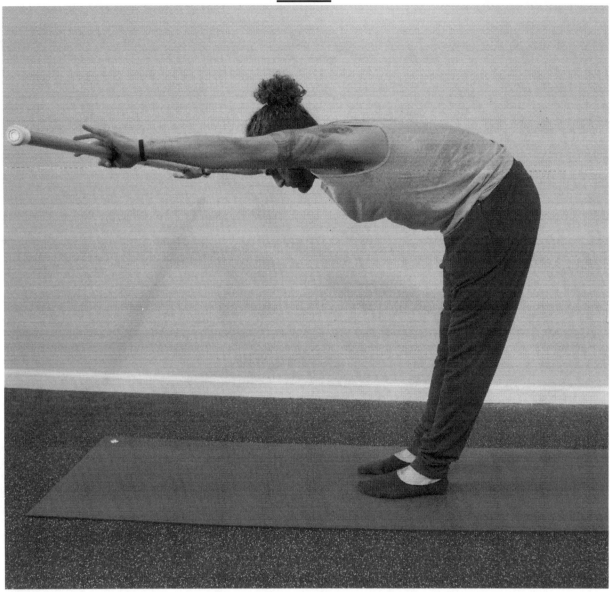

Side view

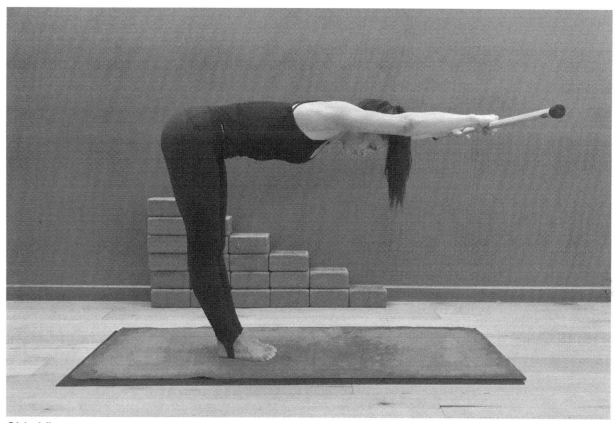

Side View

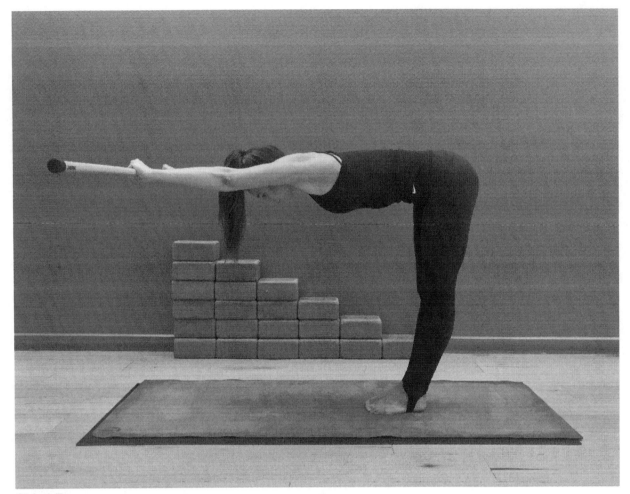
Side View

Pulsar

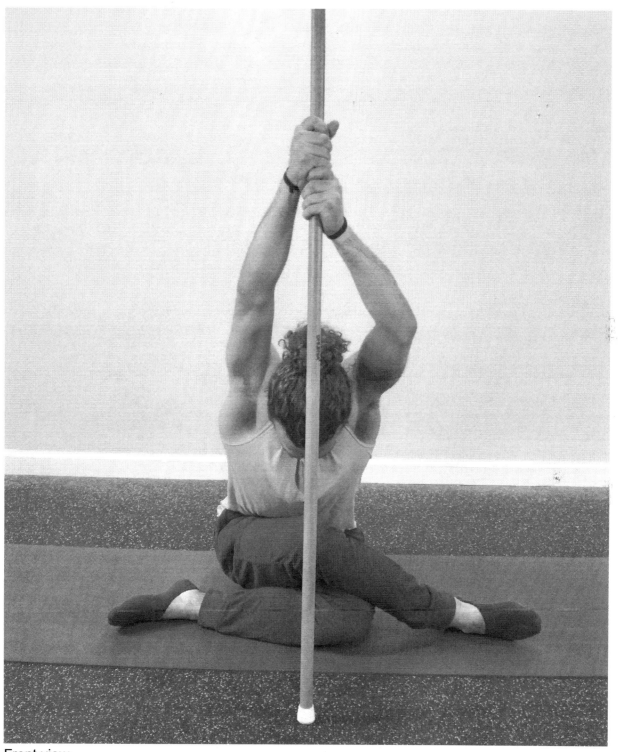

Front view

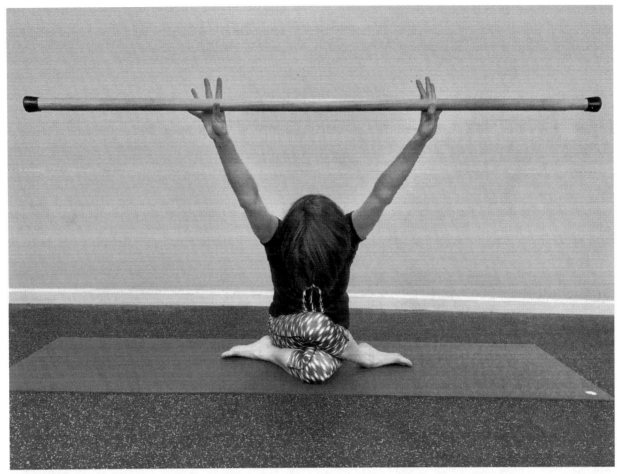

Front view

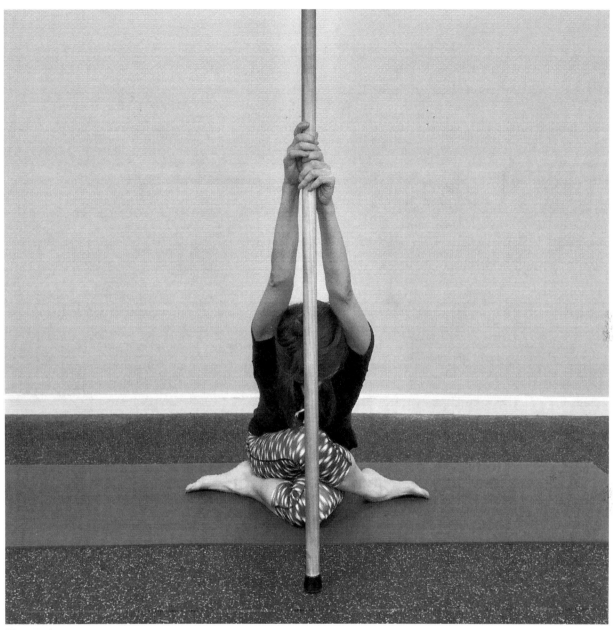

Front view

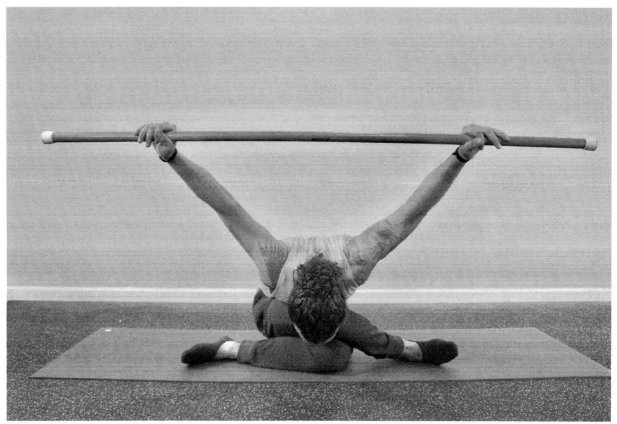

Front view

294

Pyramid

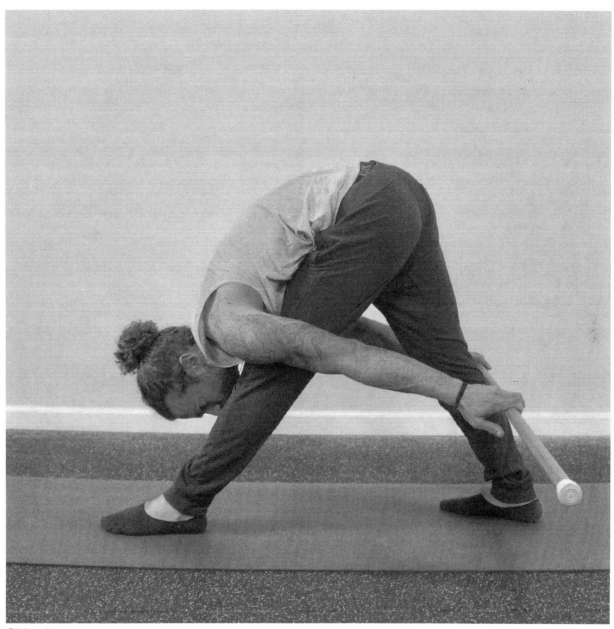

Side view

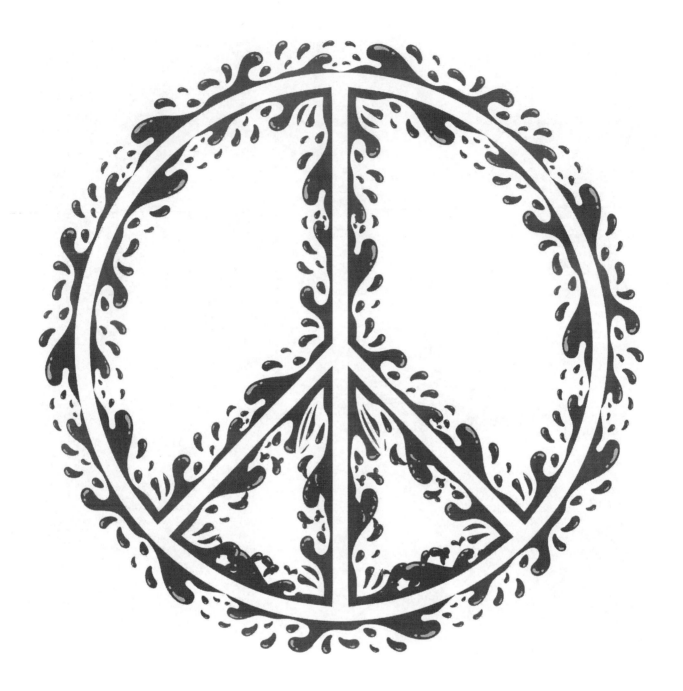

Queen L

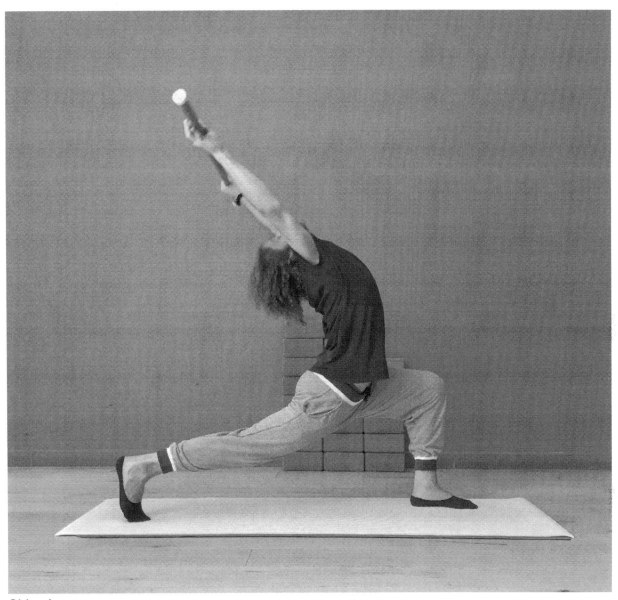

Side view

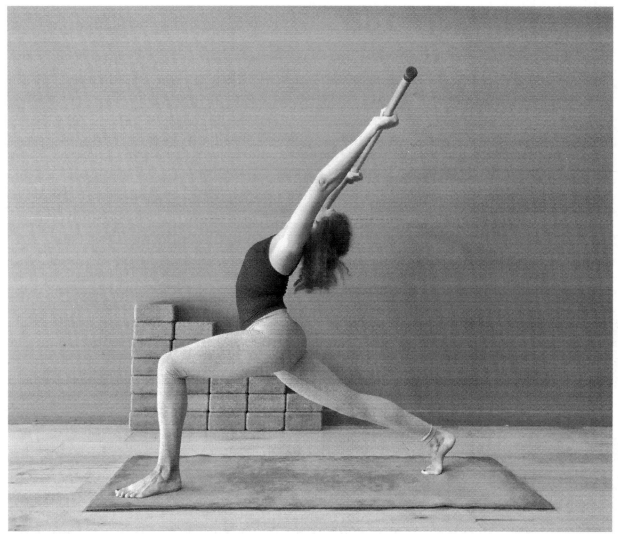
Side view

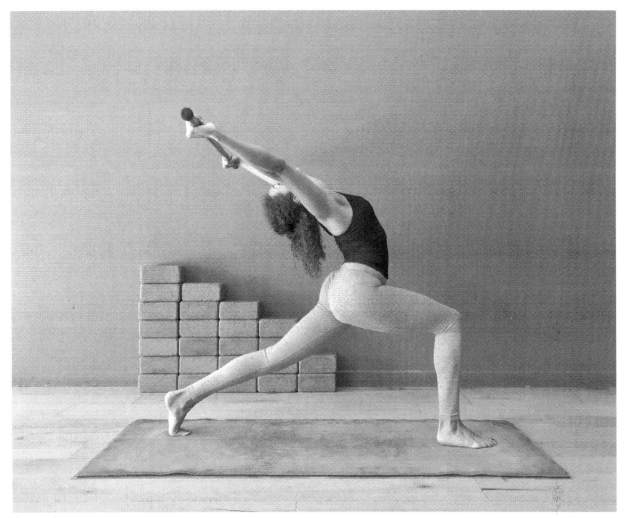

Side view

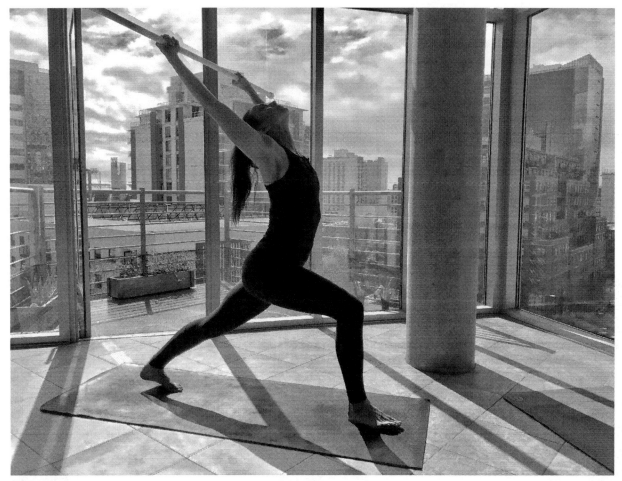
Side view

Quick

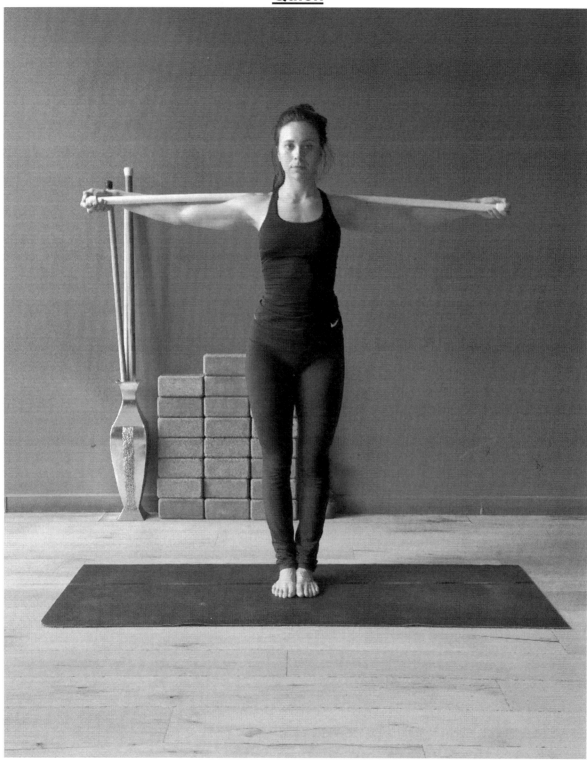

Front view

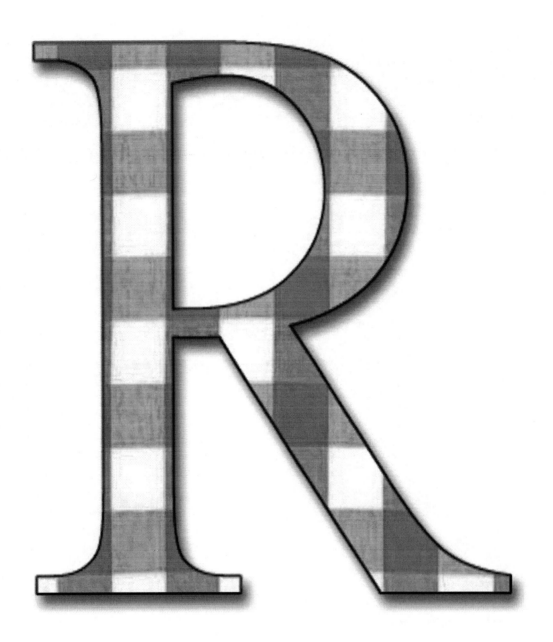

Radial

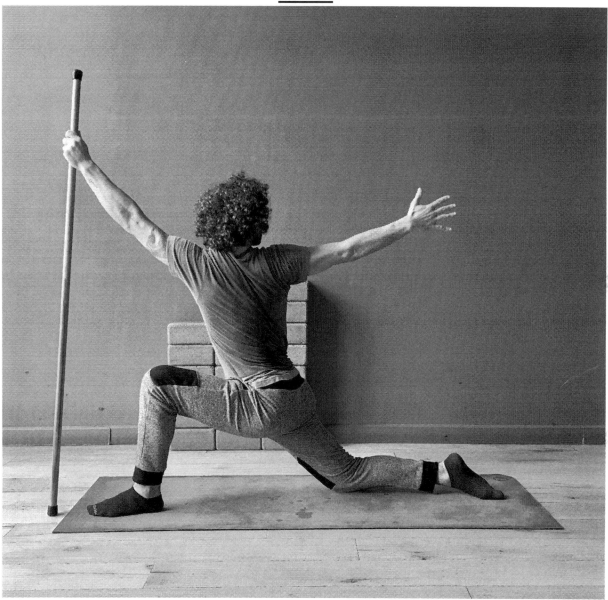

Rear Side view

Red Giant

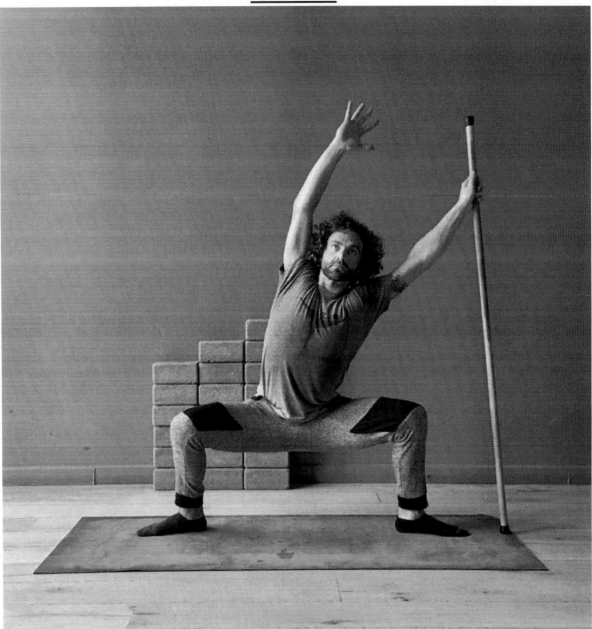

Front view

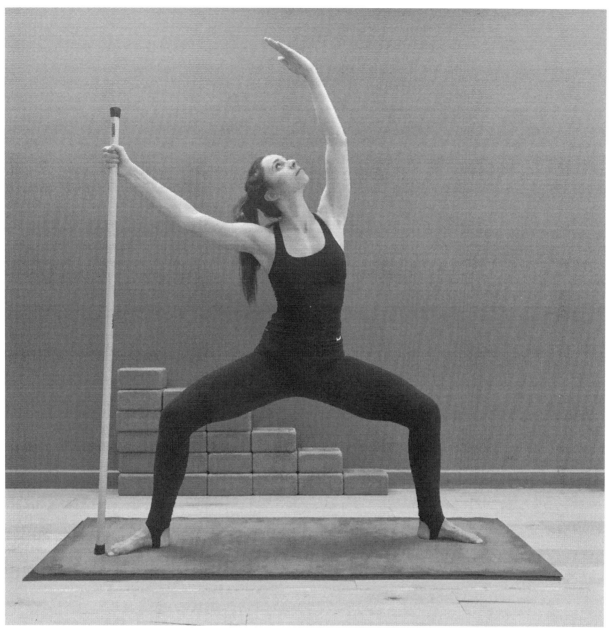
Front view

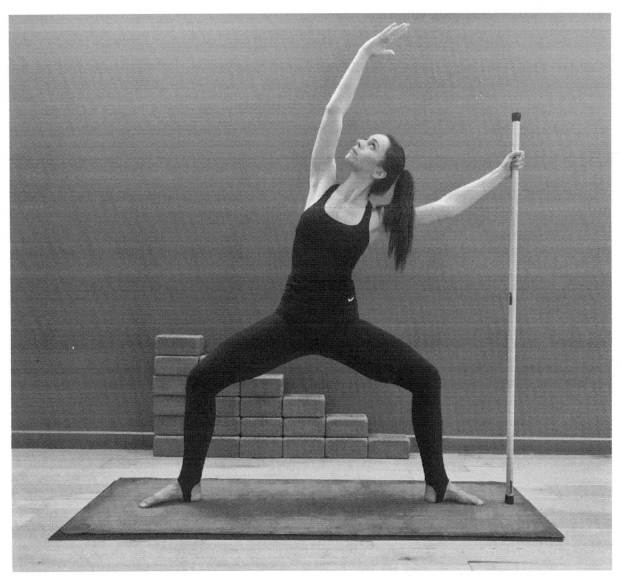

Front view

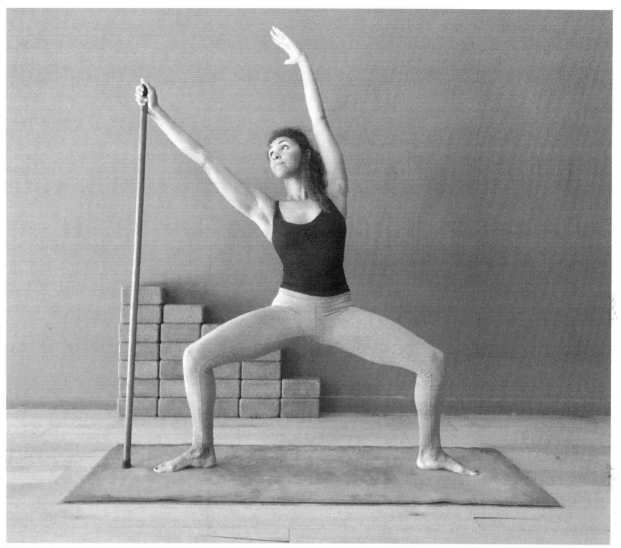

Front view

307

Reverse Triangle

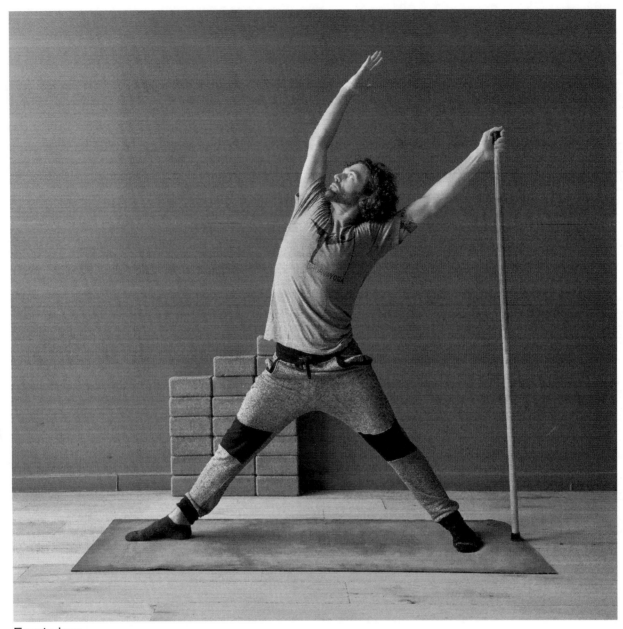
Front view

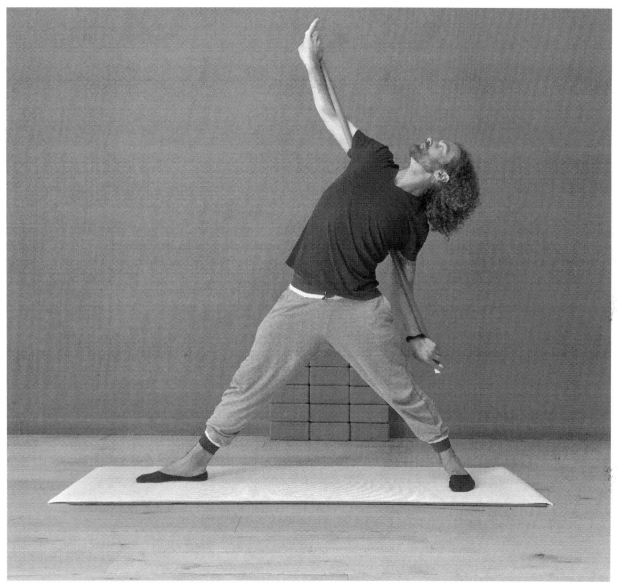

Front view

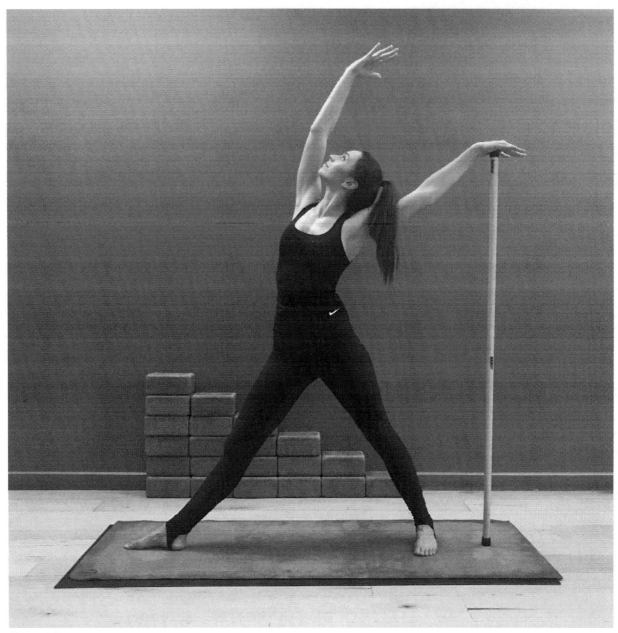

Front View

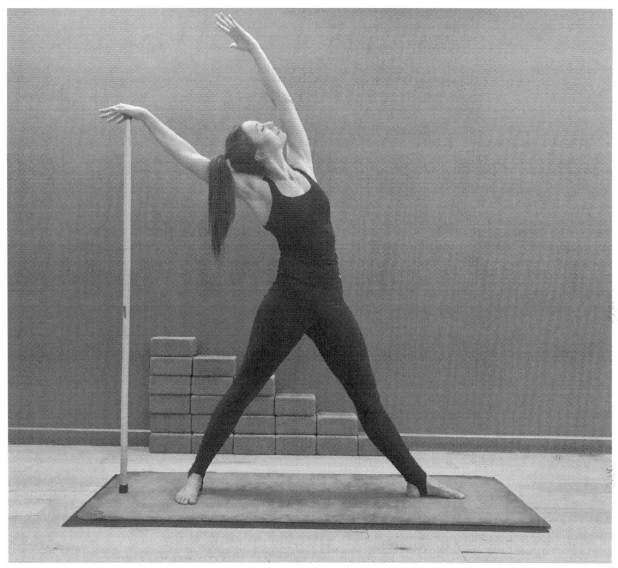

Front View

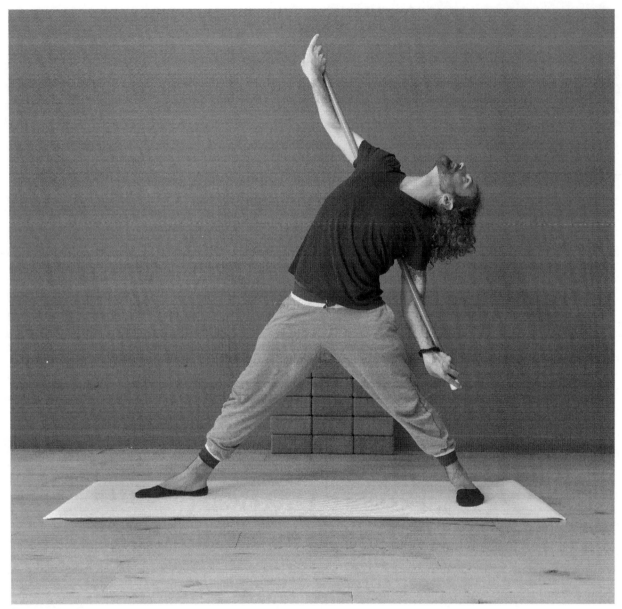

Front view

312

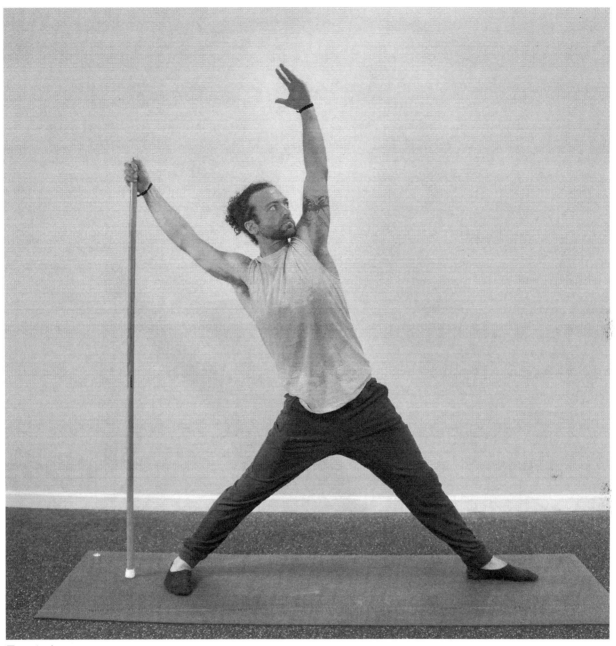

Front view

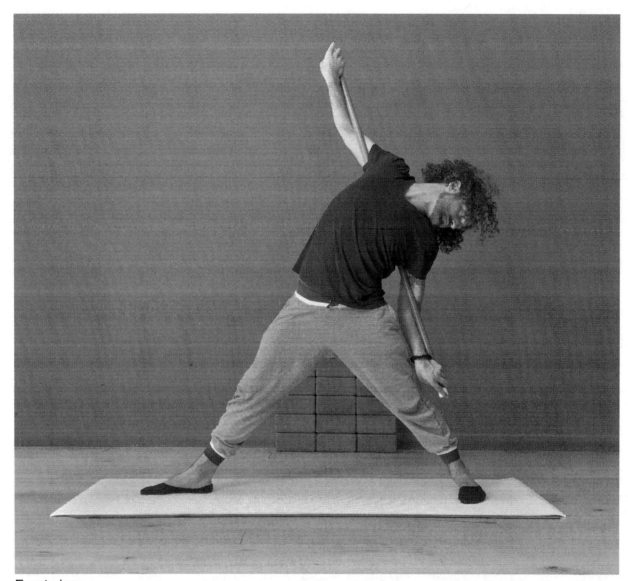

Front view

314

Reverse Warrior

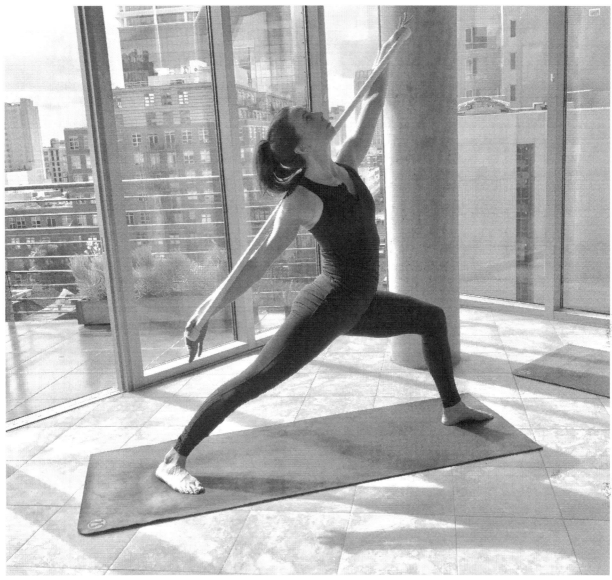

Side view

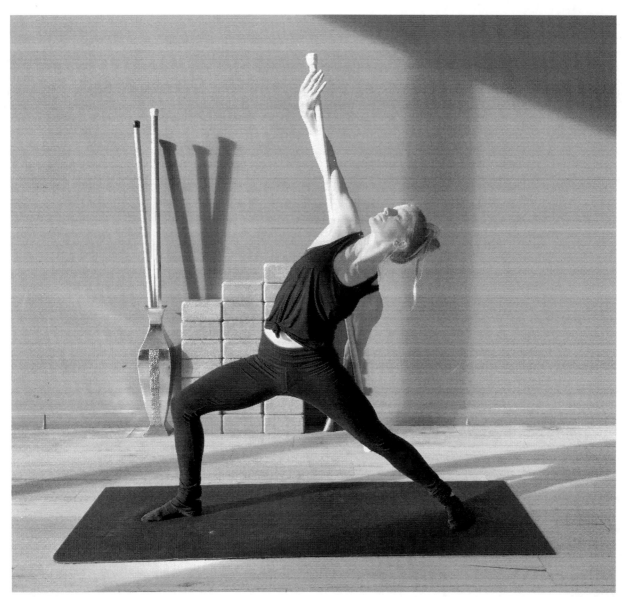

Front view

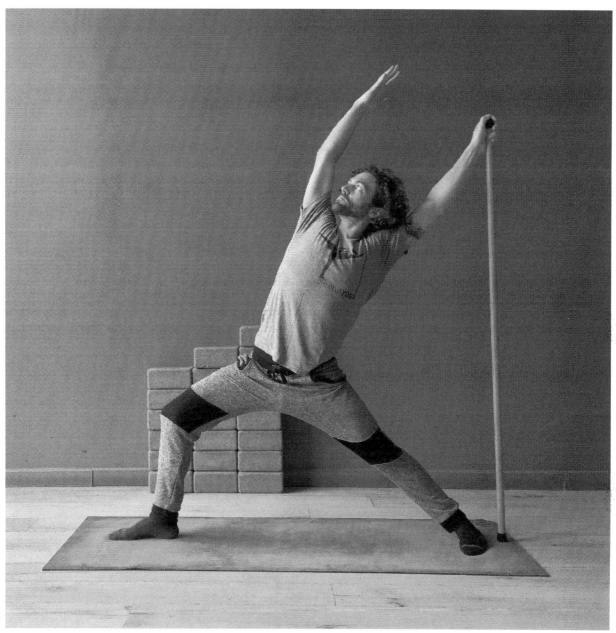

Front view

Risky

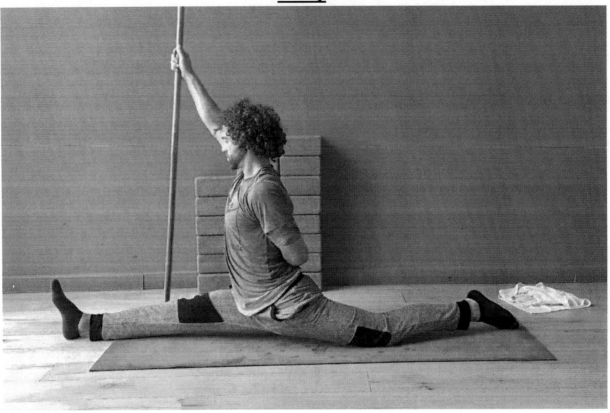

Side view

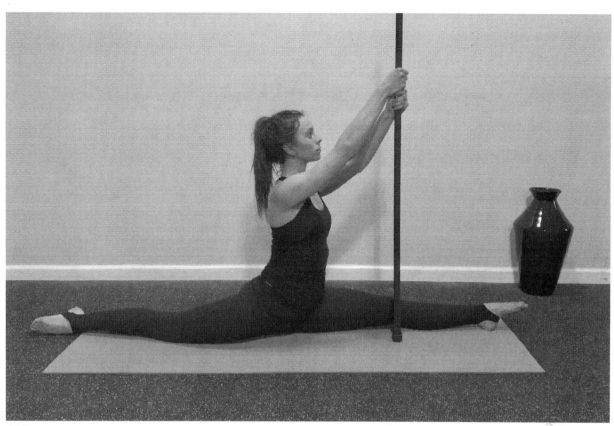
Side view

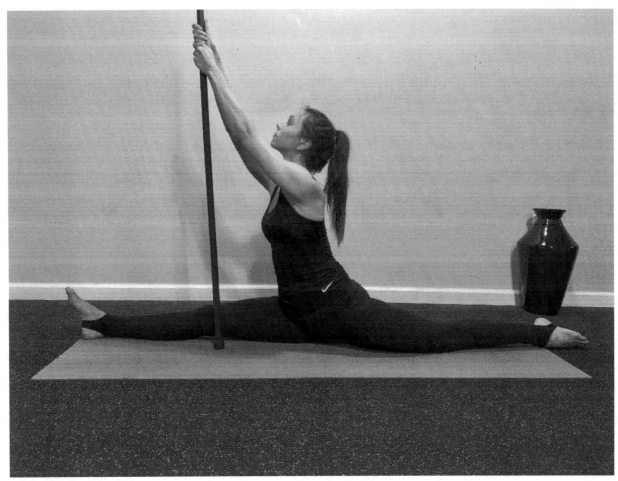

Side view

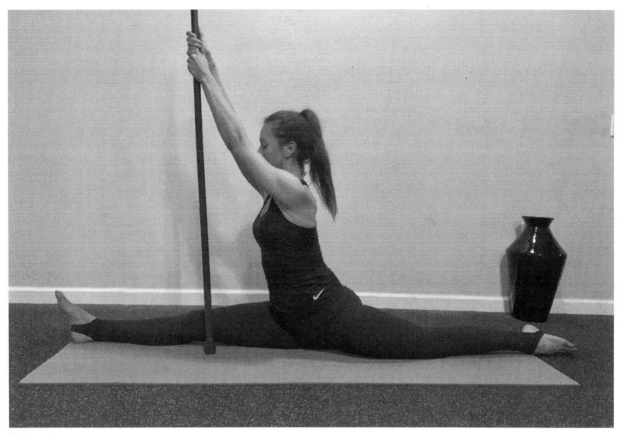
Side view

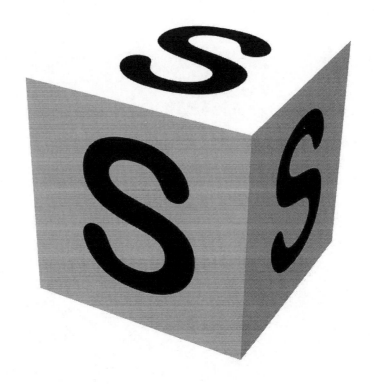

Sagittarius

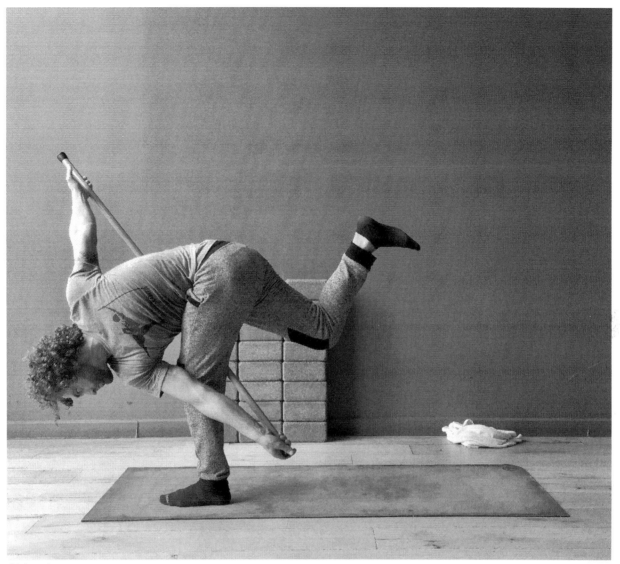

Side view

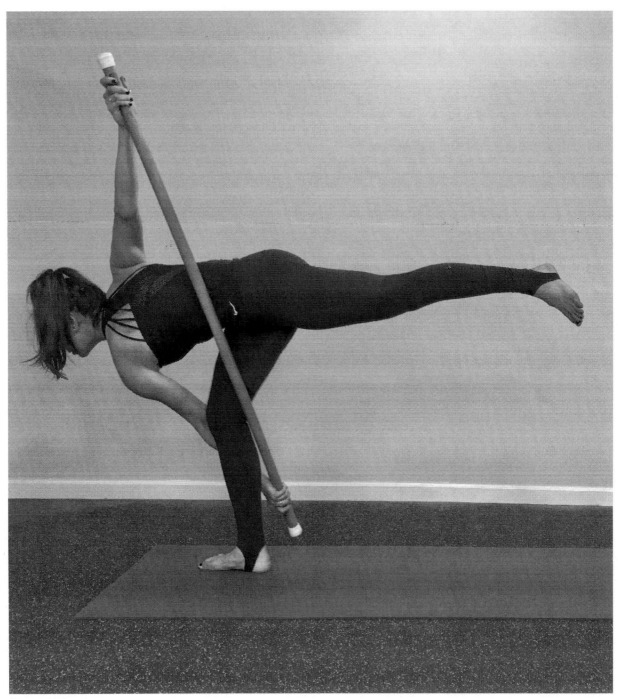

Rear Side view

Scorpio

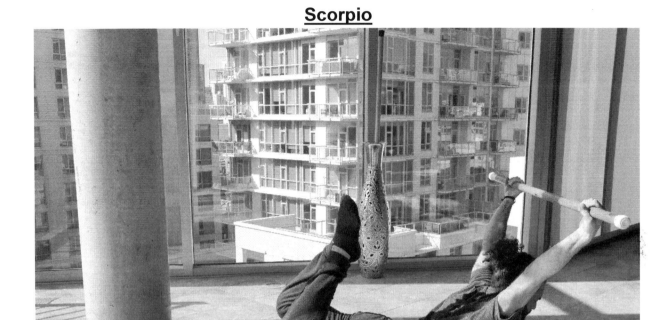

Side view

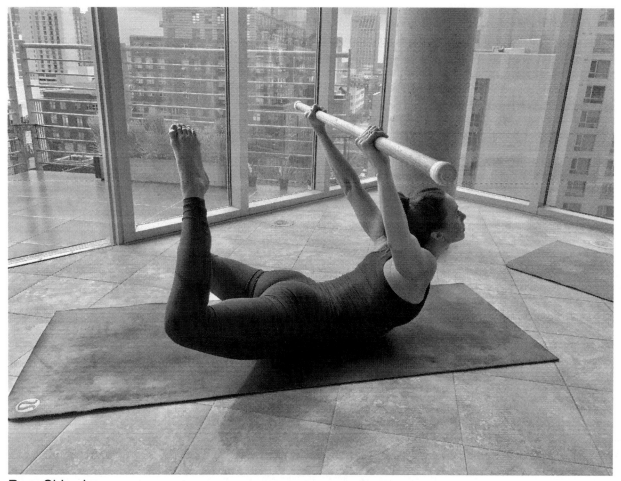

Rear Side view

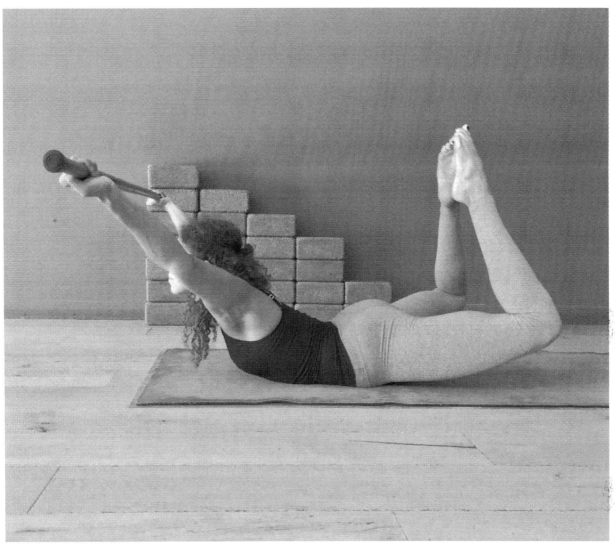

Side view

Seahorse

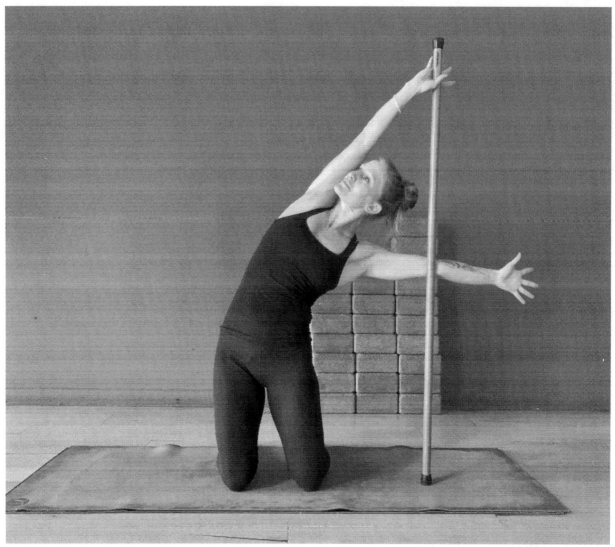

Front view

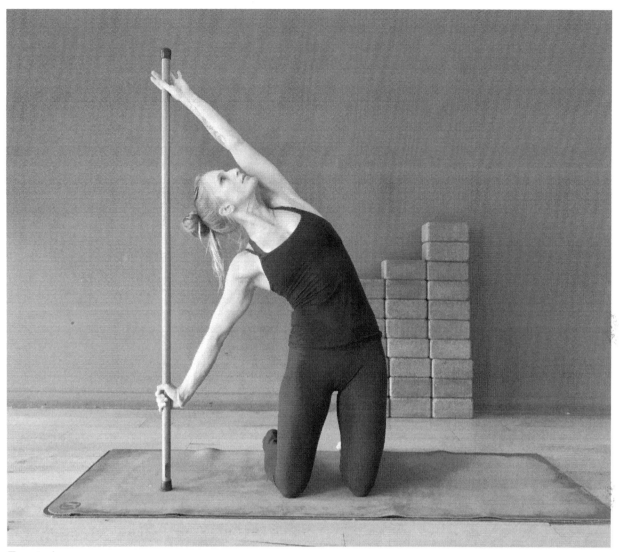

Front view

329

__Shoulder Stand__

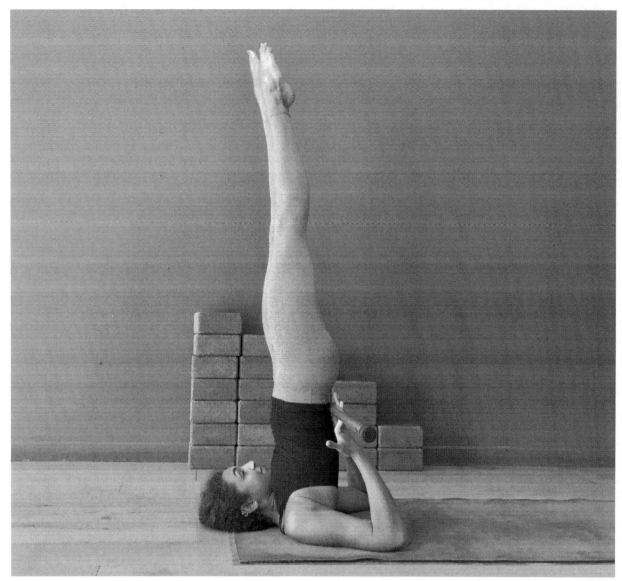

Side view

330

Side Plank

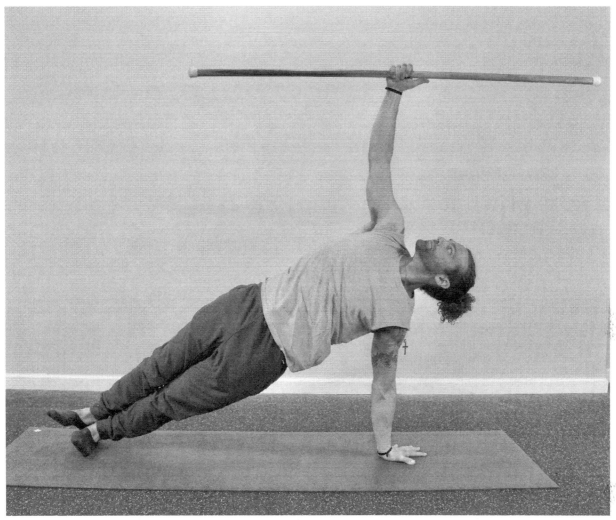
Front view

Side Star

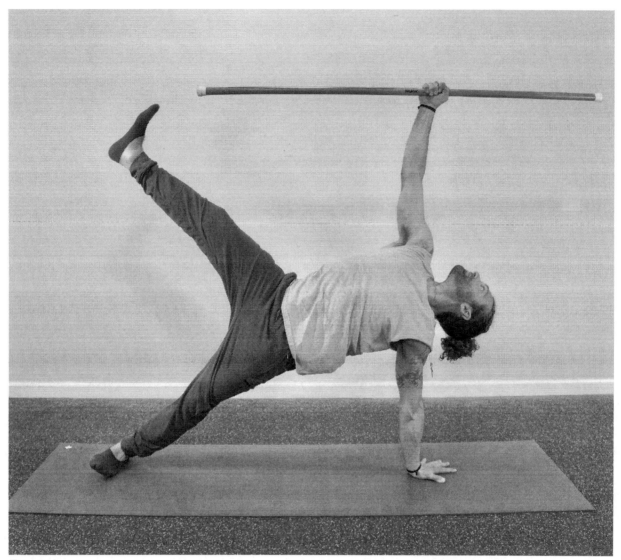
Front view

Smile

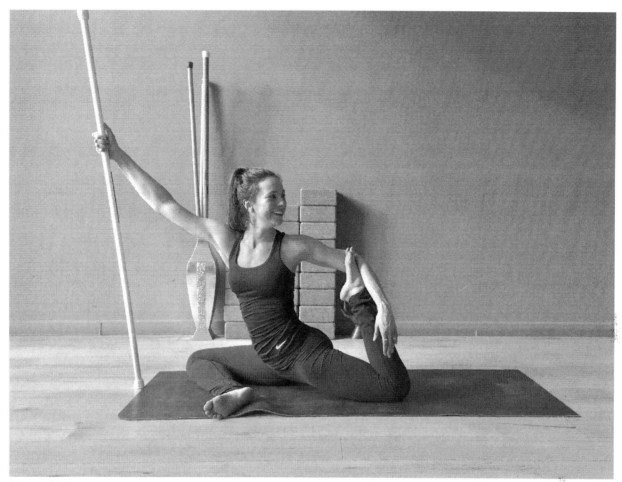

Front Side view

Solar Flare

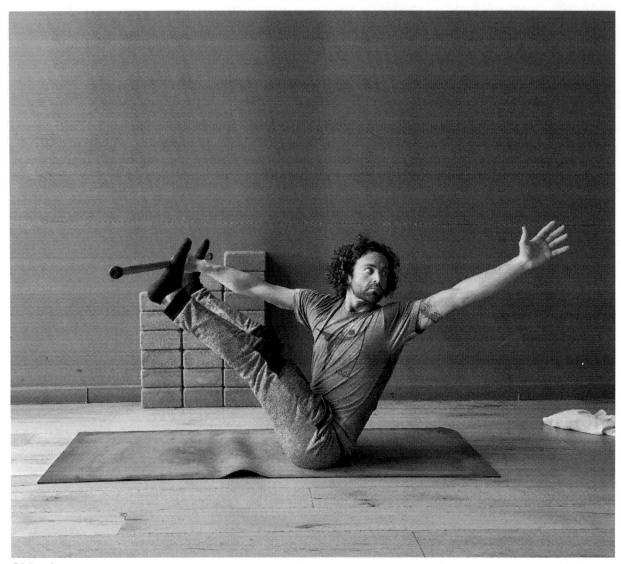

Side view

334

<u>Solstice</u>

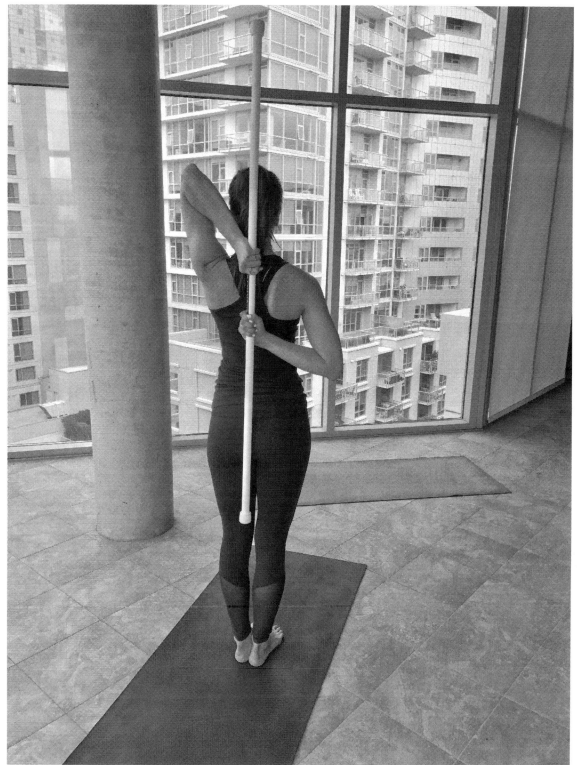

Rear view

Spectrum

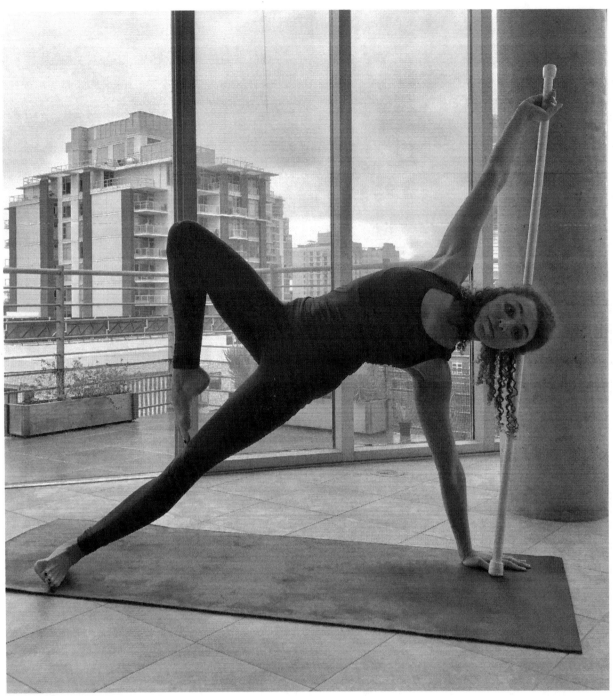

Front view

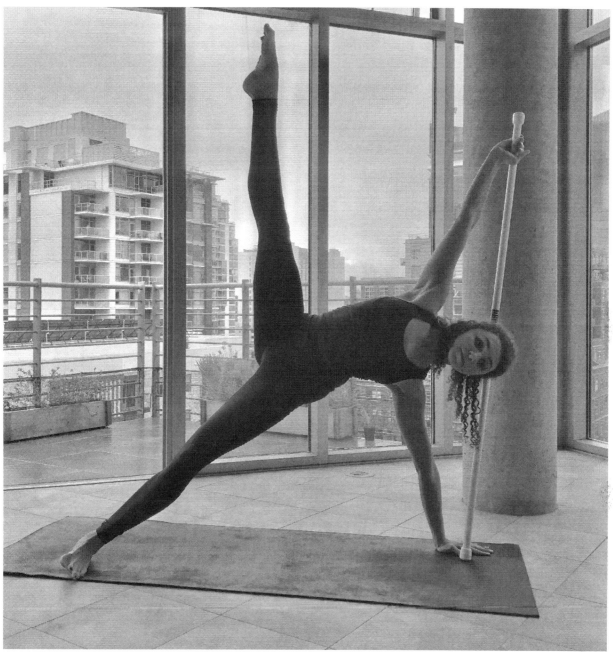
Front view

Sprinter

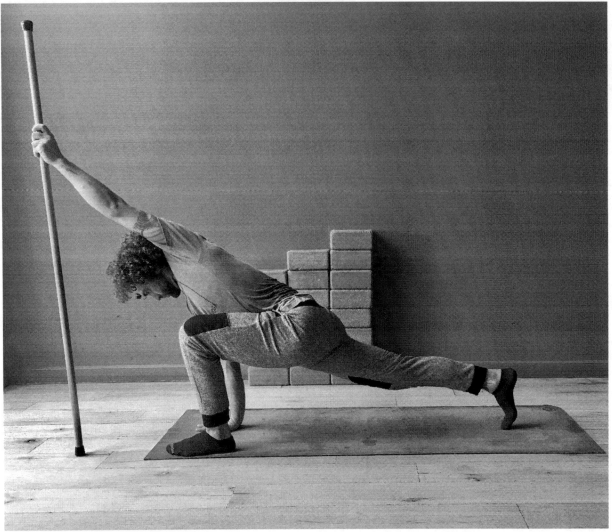

Side view

Sponge

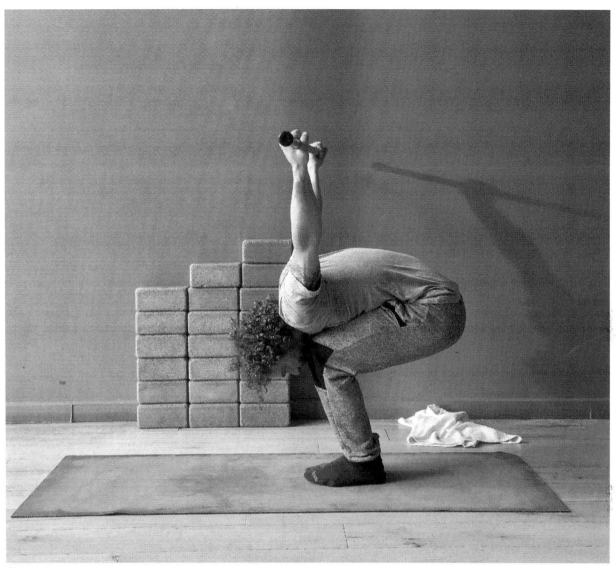

Side view

SSLFK

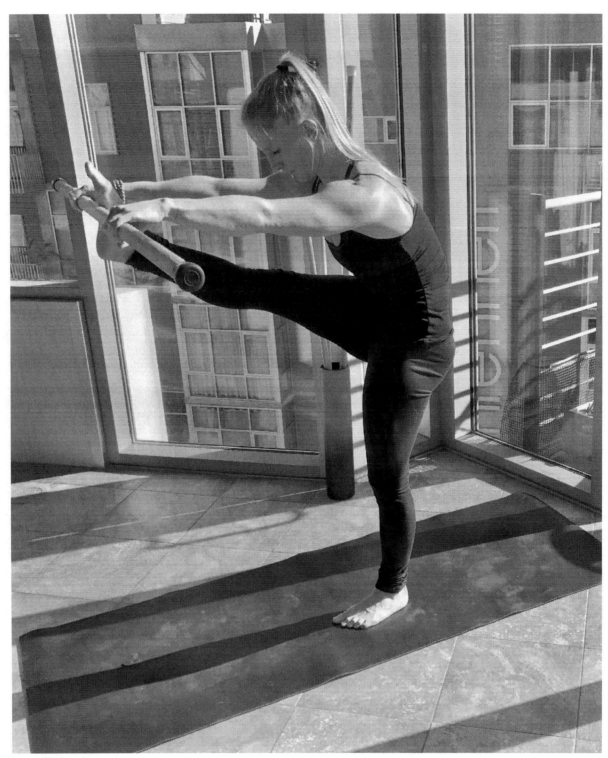

Front Side view

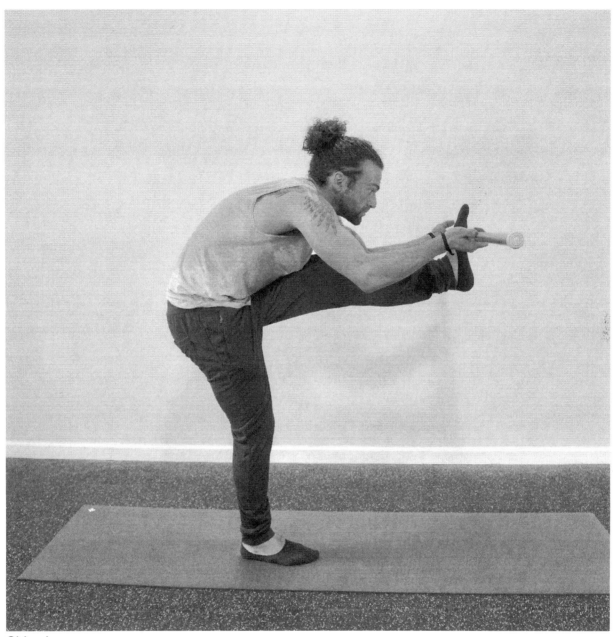

Side view

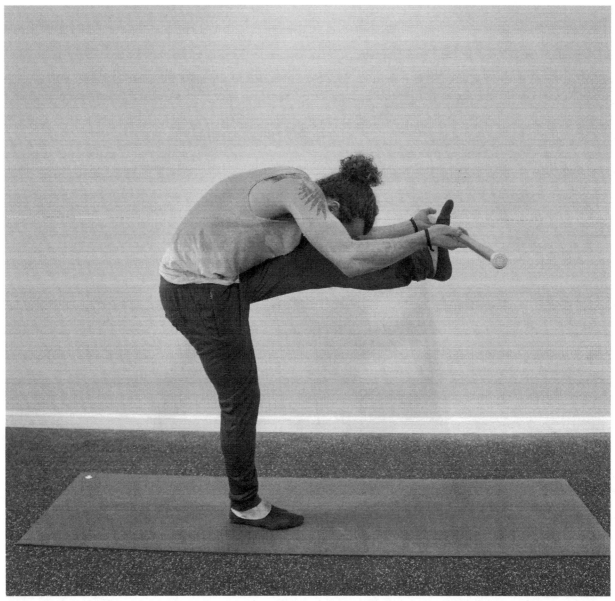

Side view

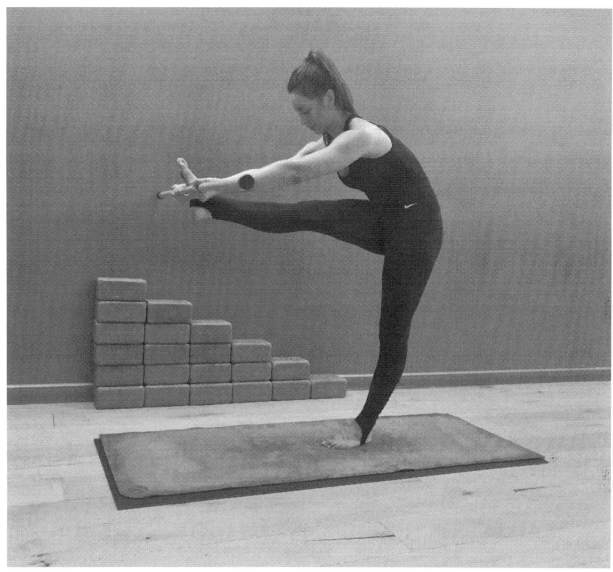

Front Side view

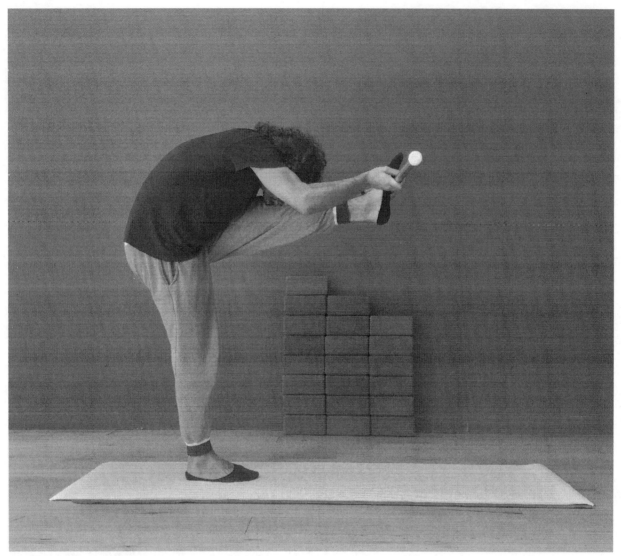

Side view

Standing Splits

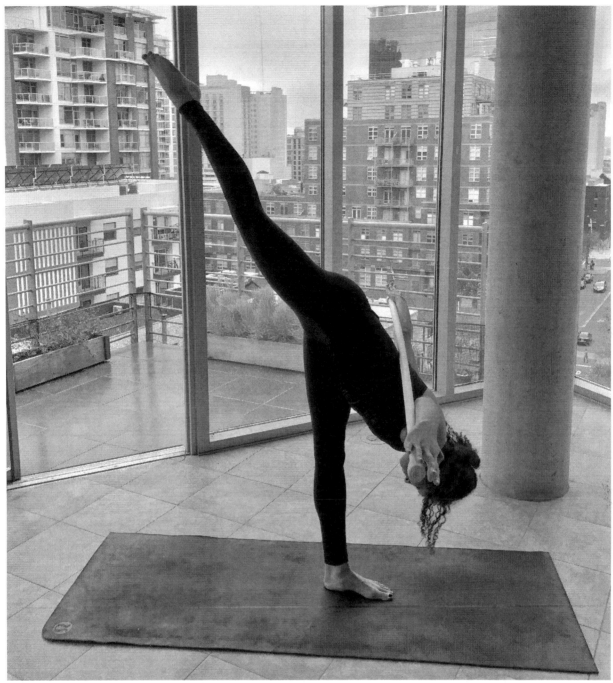

Side view

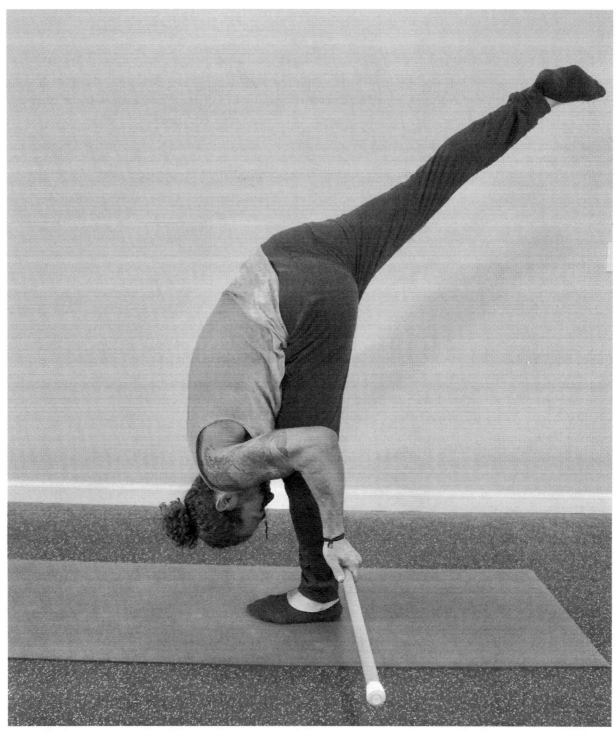
Side view

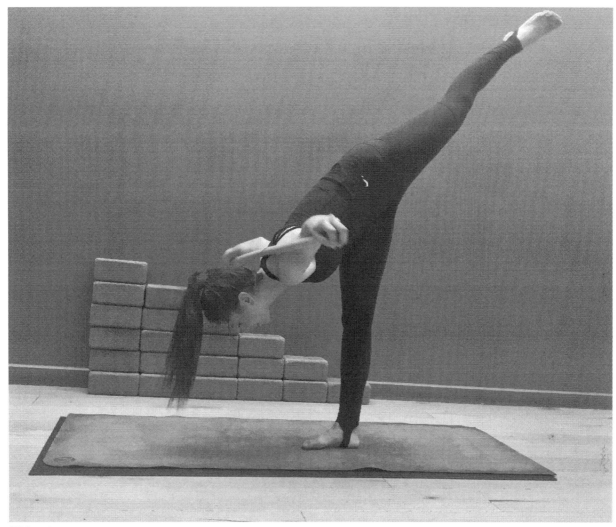

Side view

Sunspot

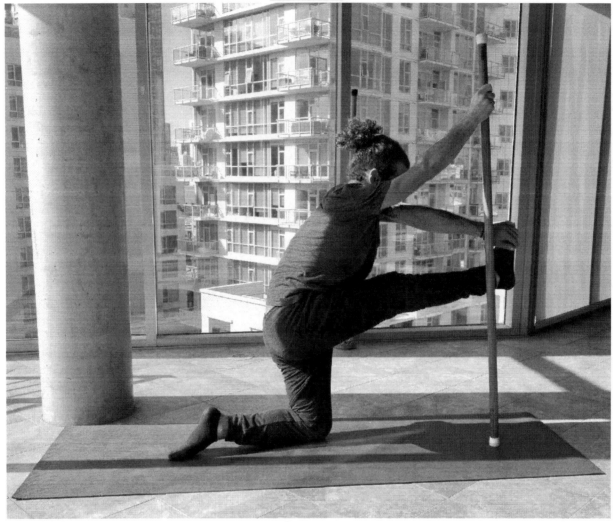

Side view

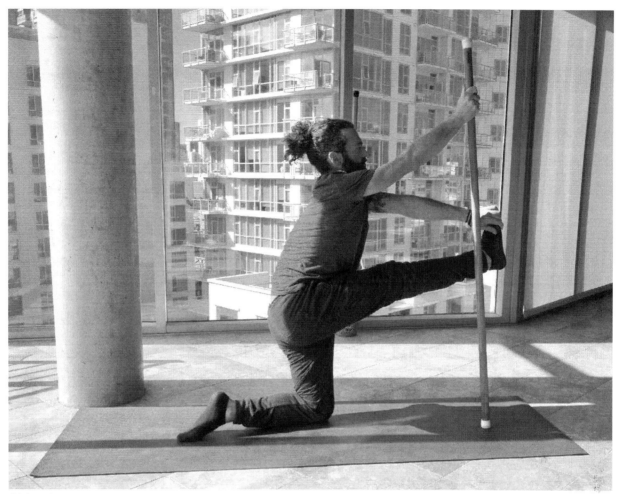

Side view

Super Moon

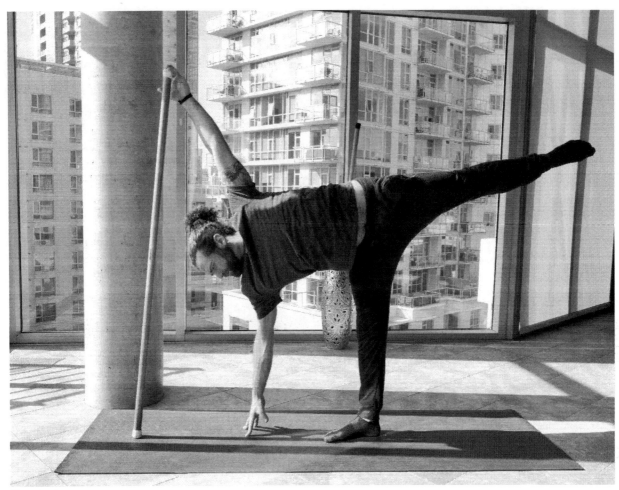

Front view

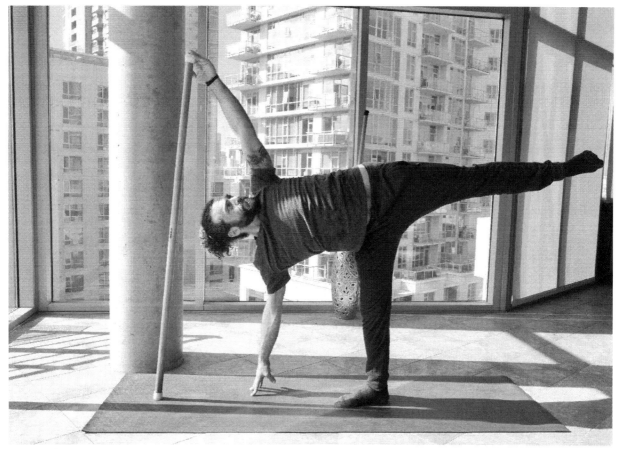

Front view

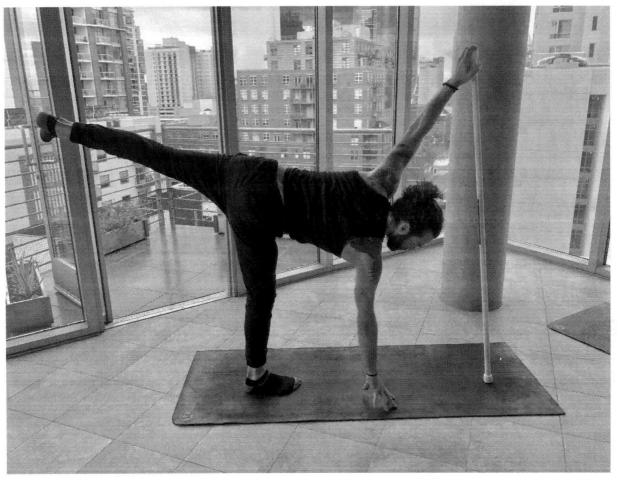

Rear view

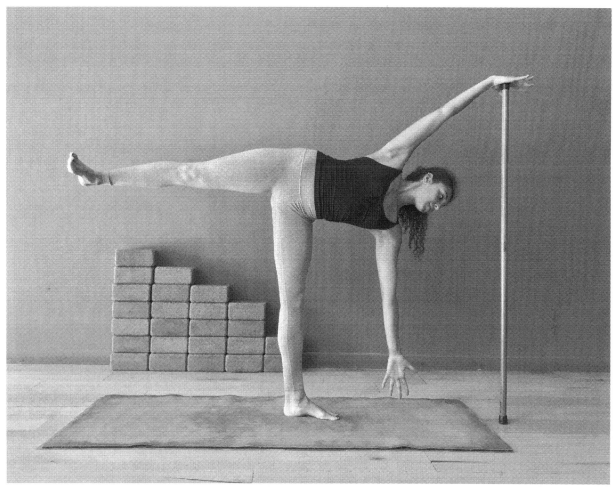
Front view

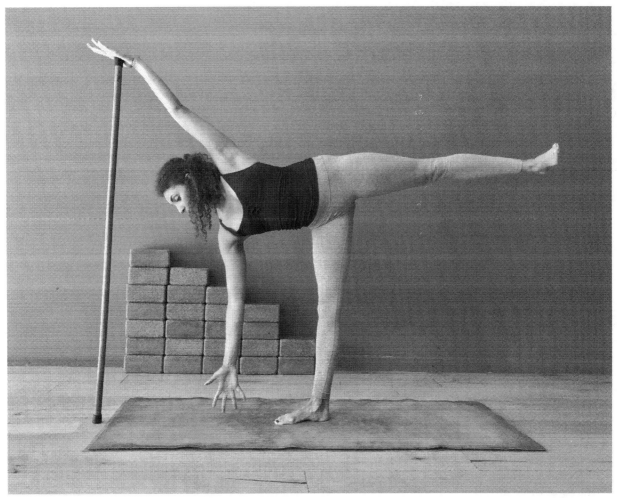
Front view

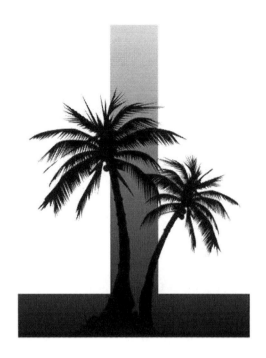

Teacher

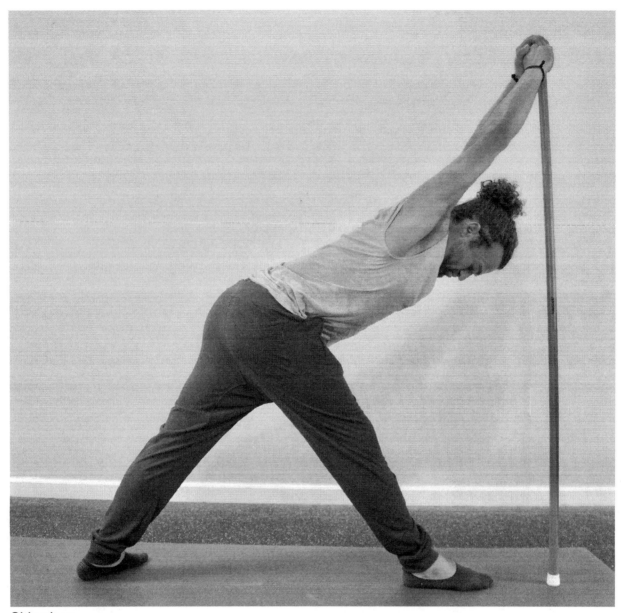

Side view

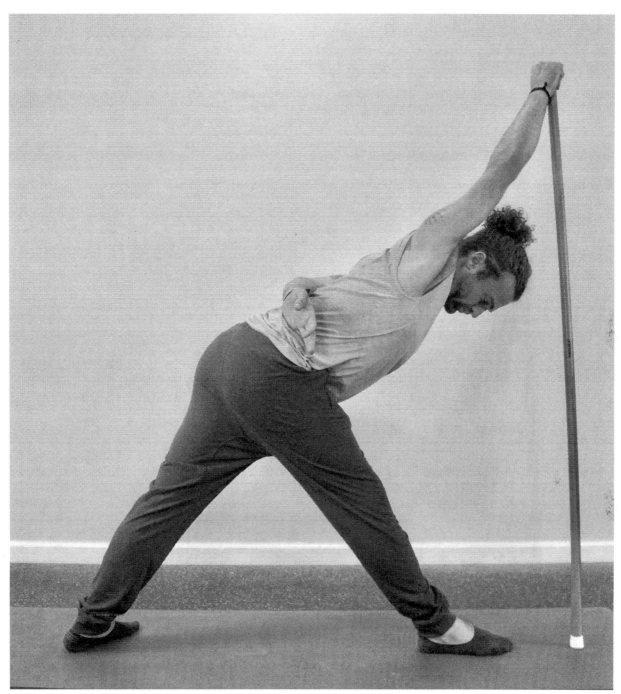

Side view

Terrestrial

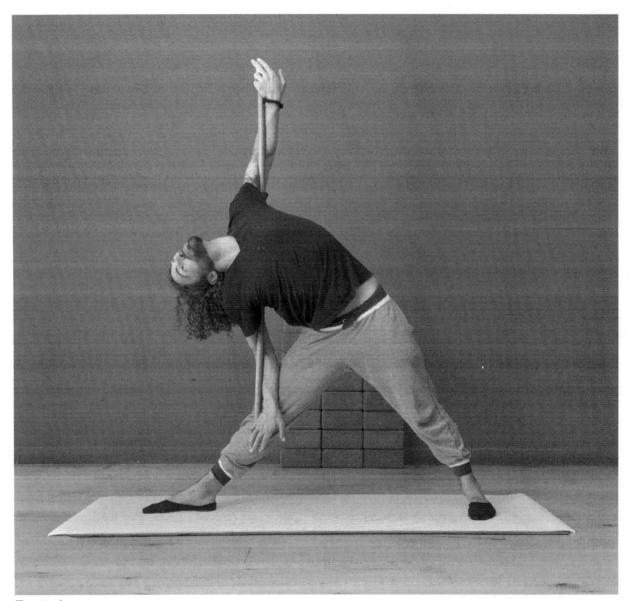

Front view

358

Tiptoe

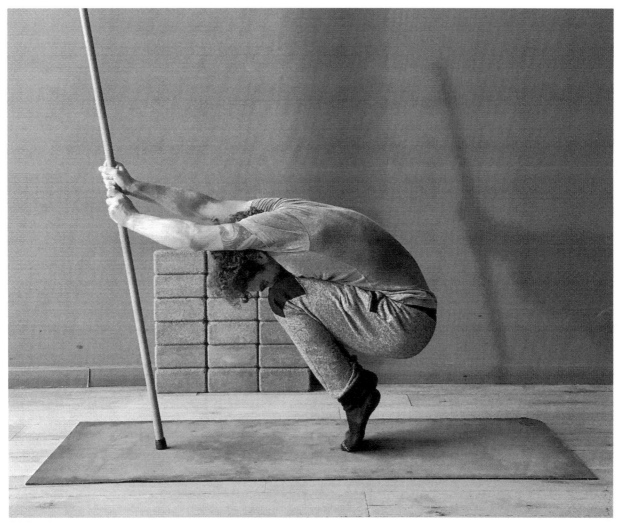

Side view

359

Tree

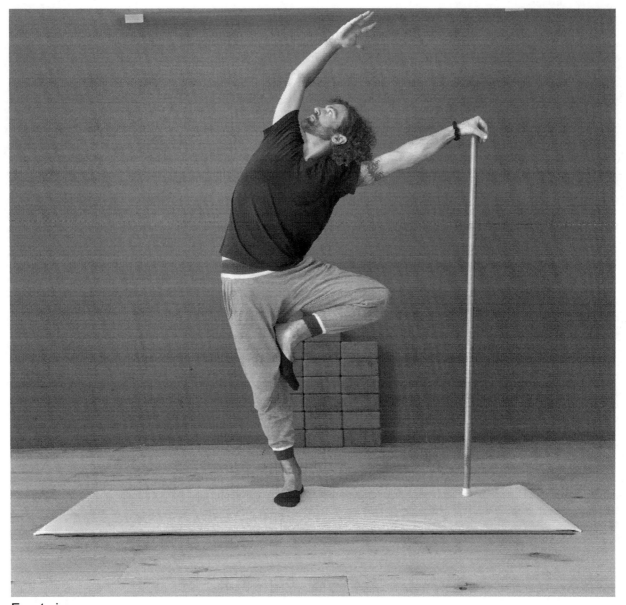

Front view

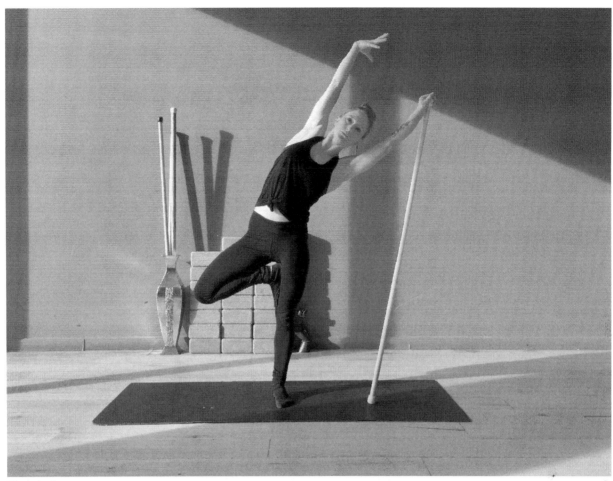
Front view

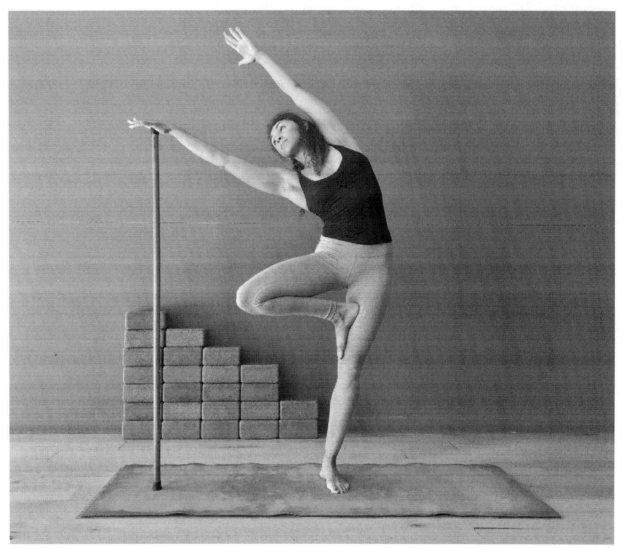

Front view

Tree Frog

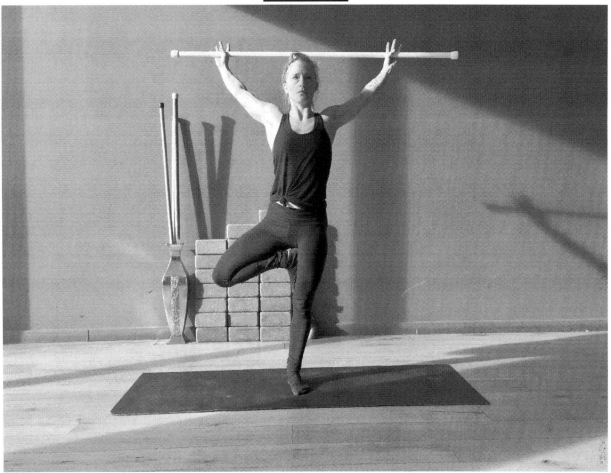

Front view

Tree Top

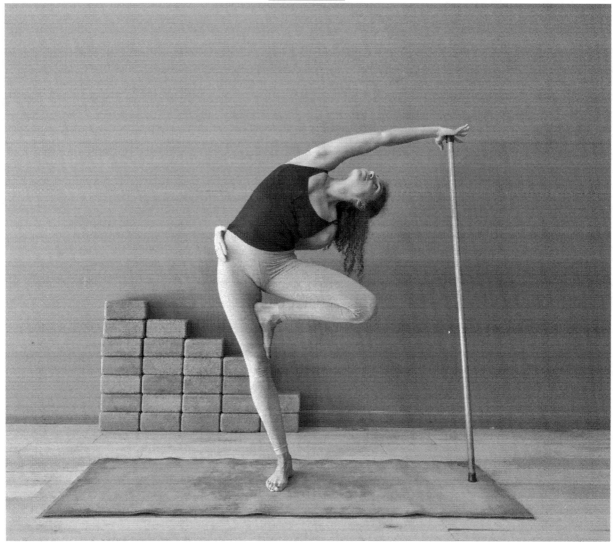

Front view

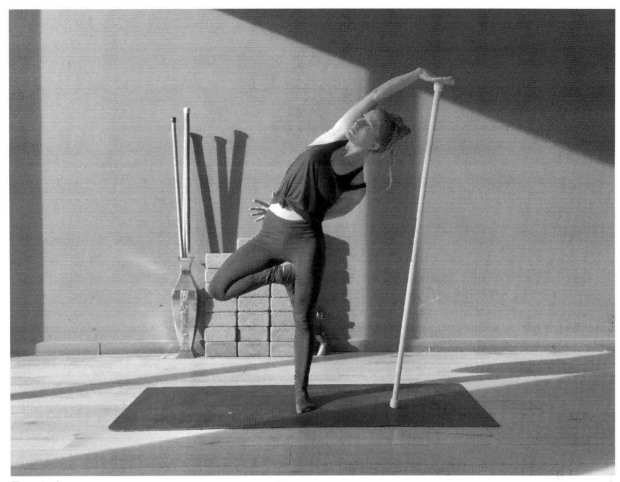

Front view

Triangle

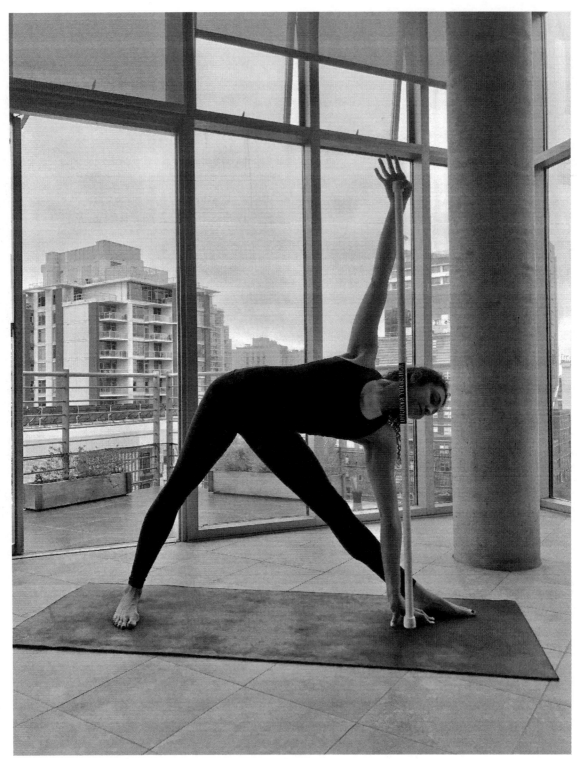

Front view

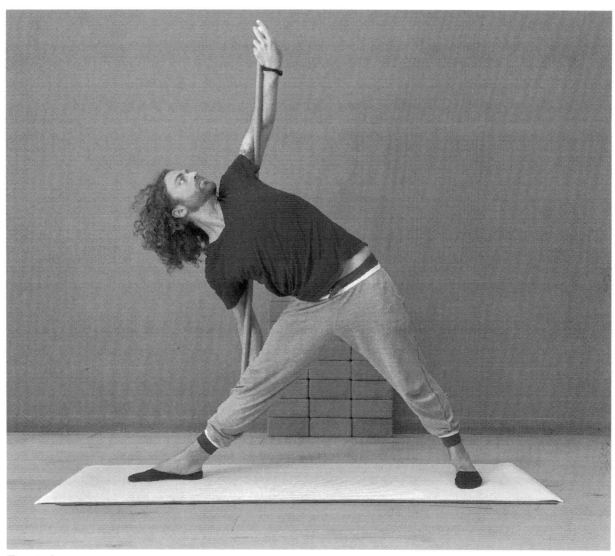

Front view

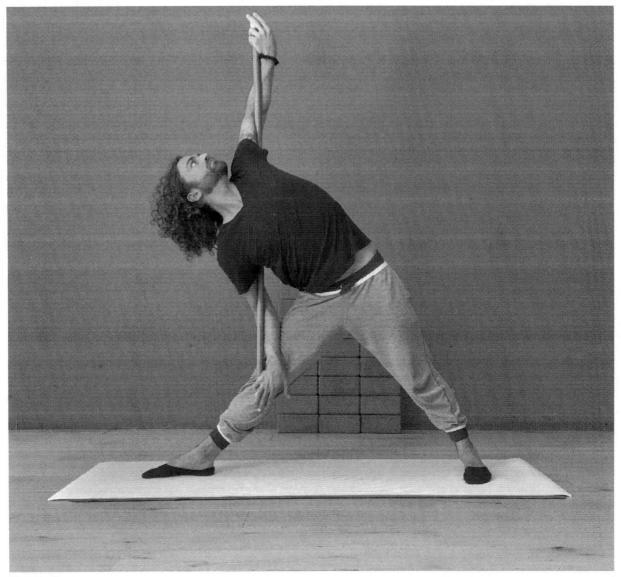

Front view

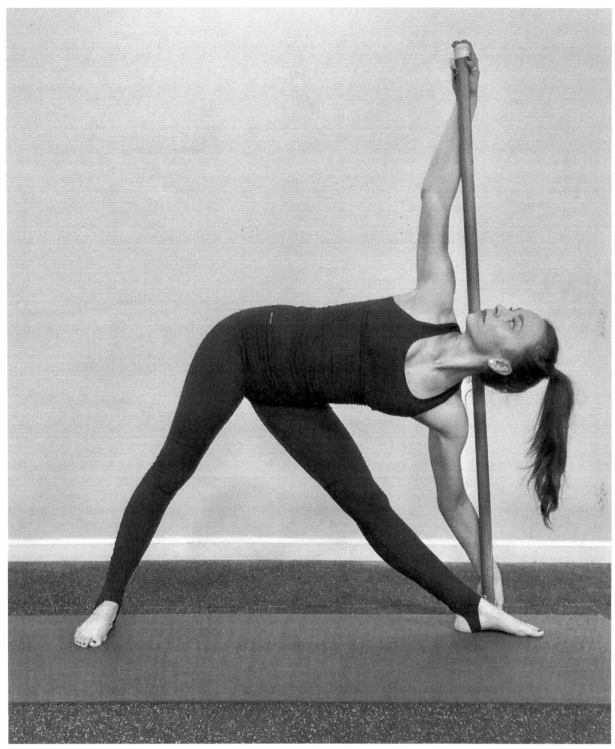

Front view

Trojan

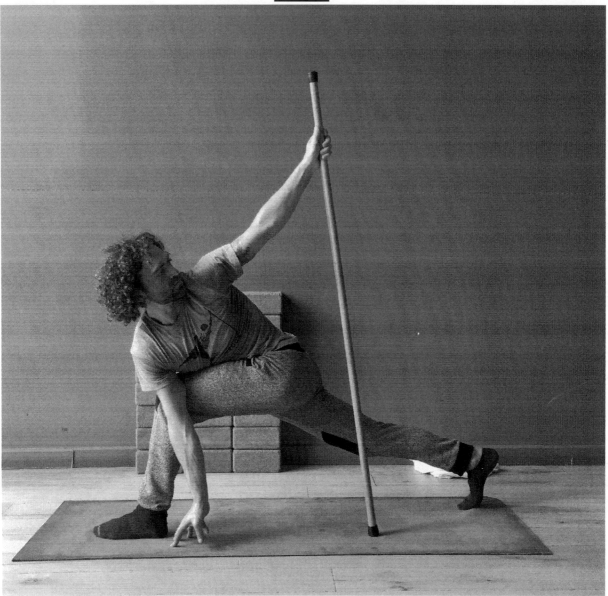

Side view

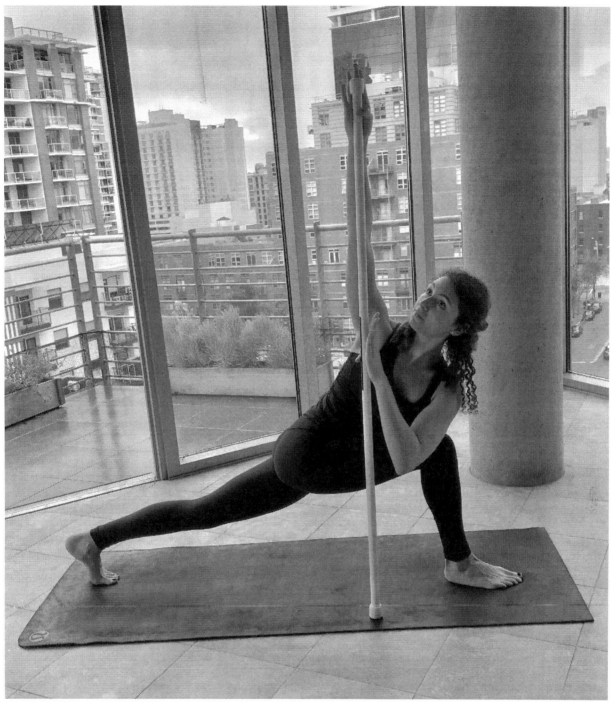
Side view

Tsunami

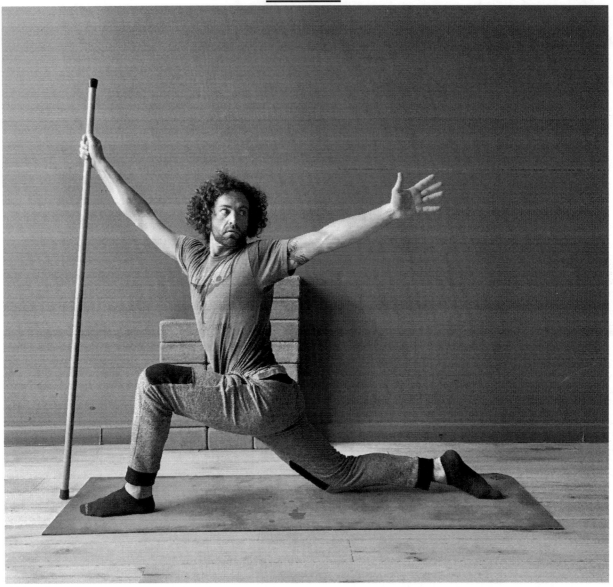

Side view

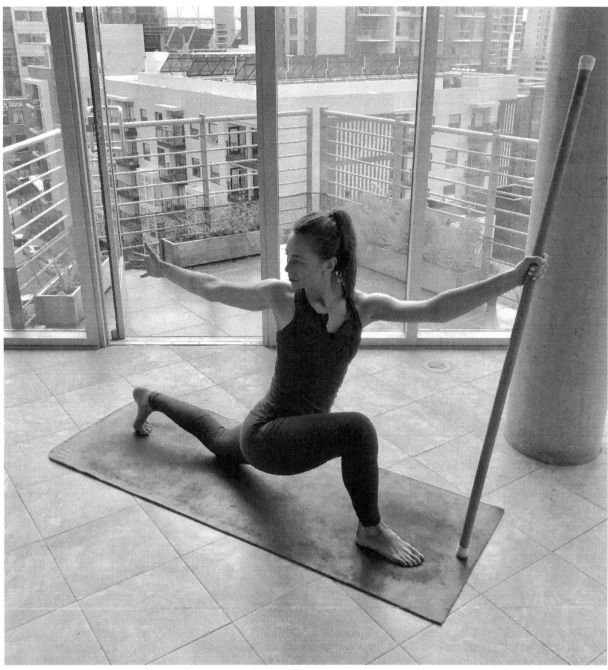

Front Side view

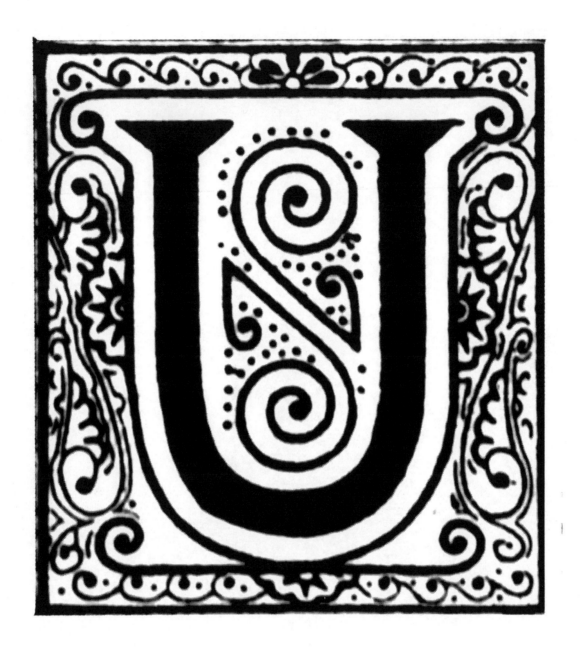

Umbra

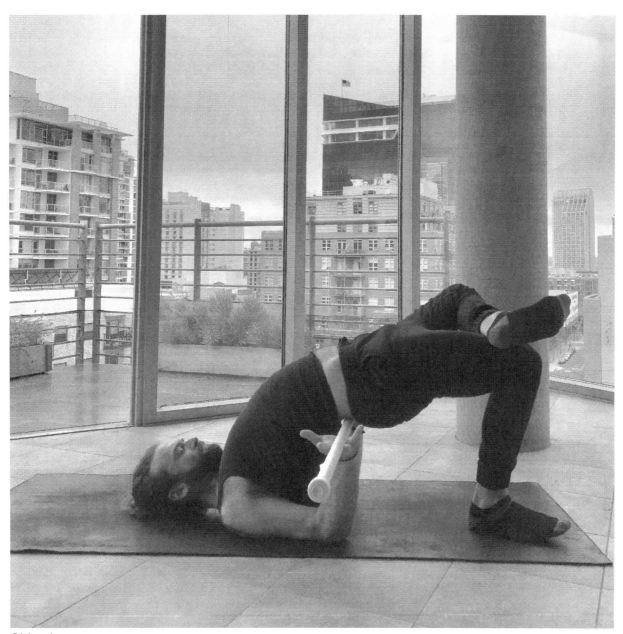

Side view

Unicorn

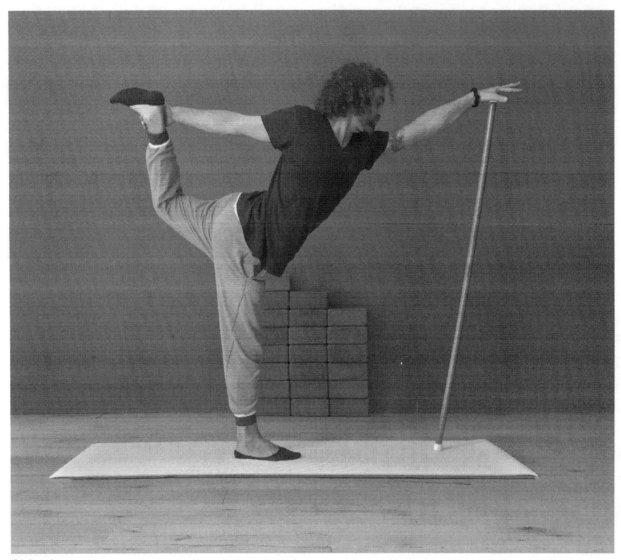
Side view

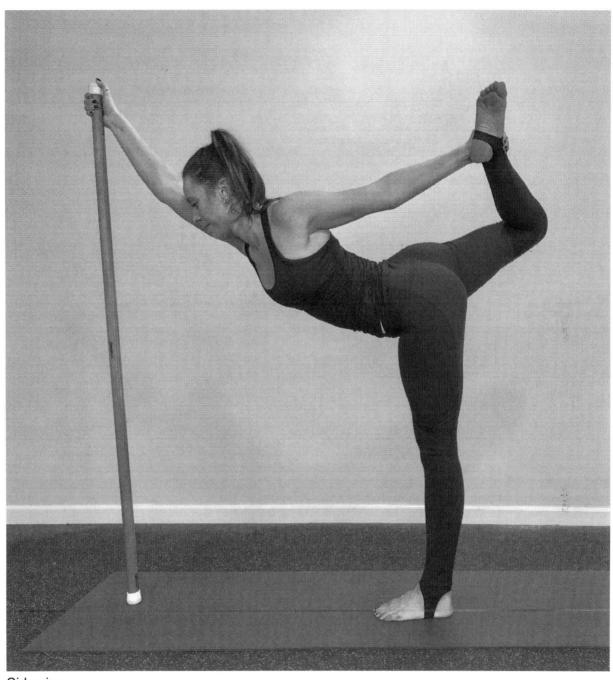

Side view

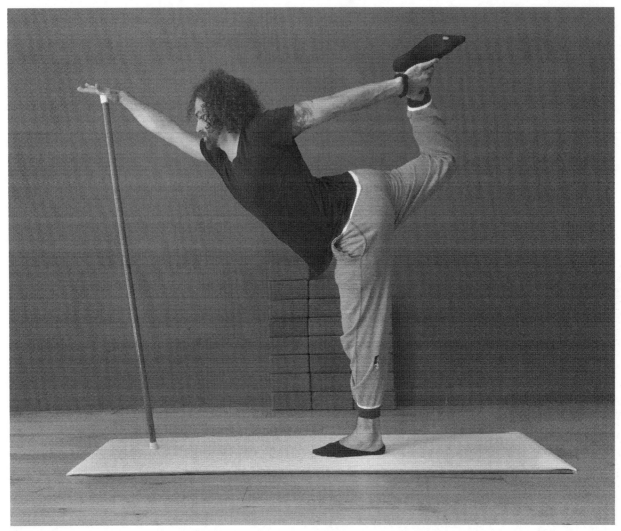

Side view

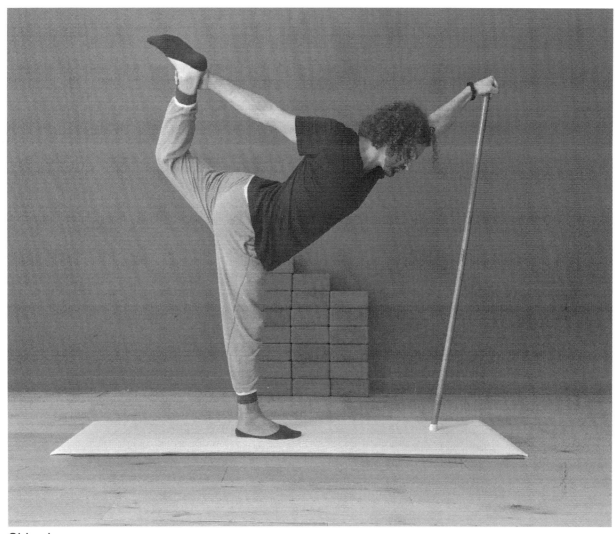

Side view

Up dog

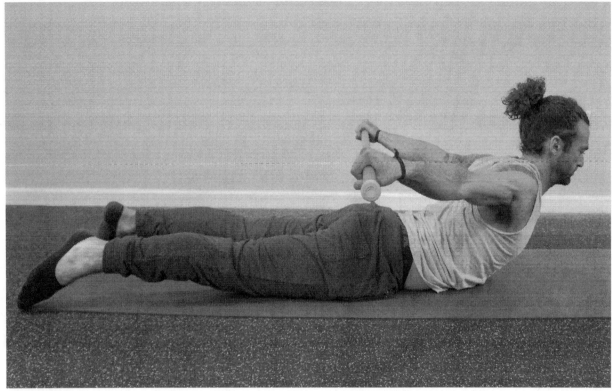

Side view

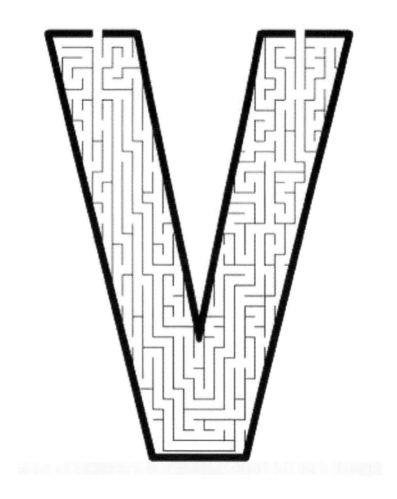

Volcano

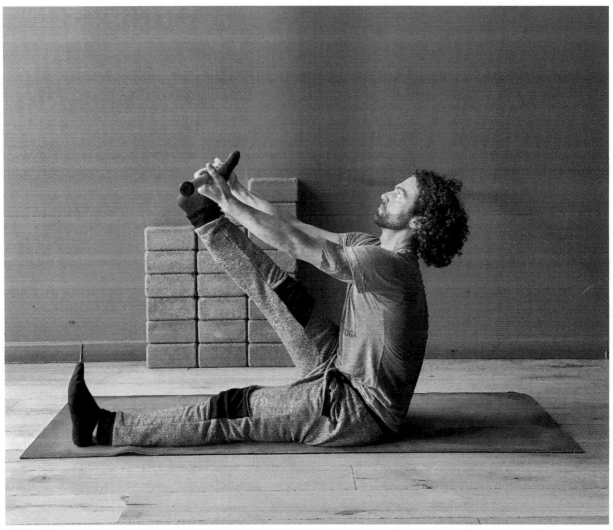
Side view

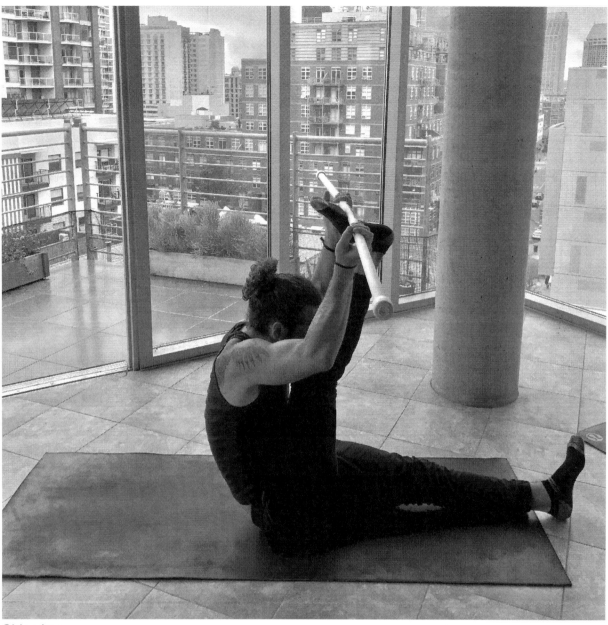

Side view

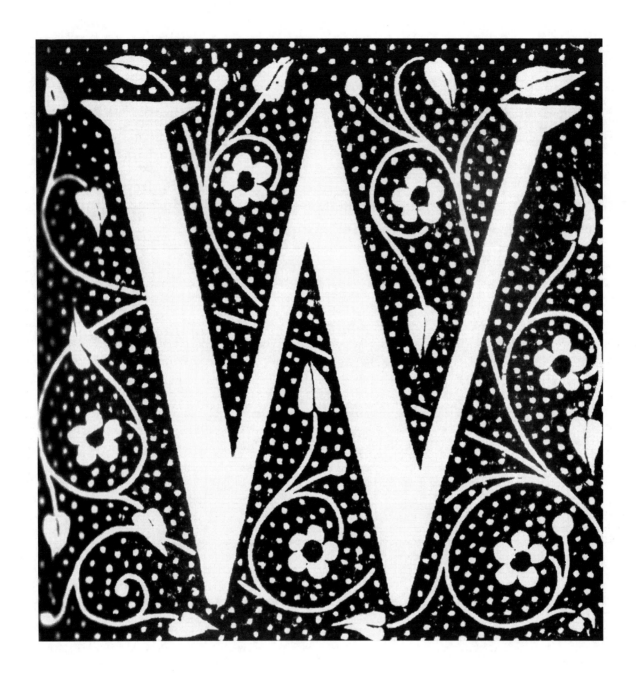

Warrior I

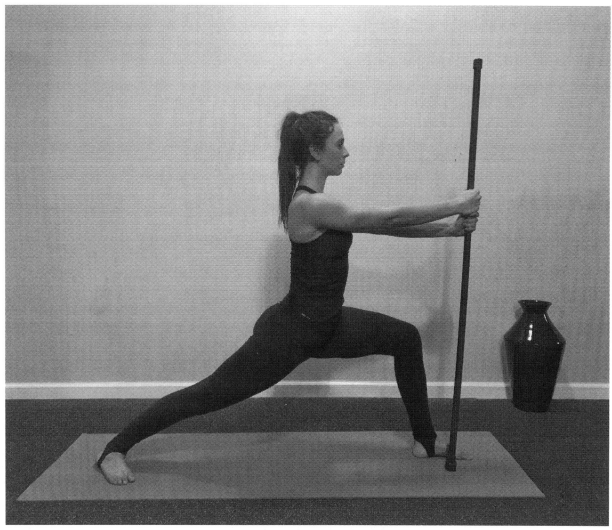

Side view

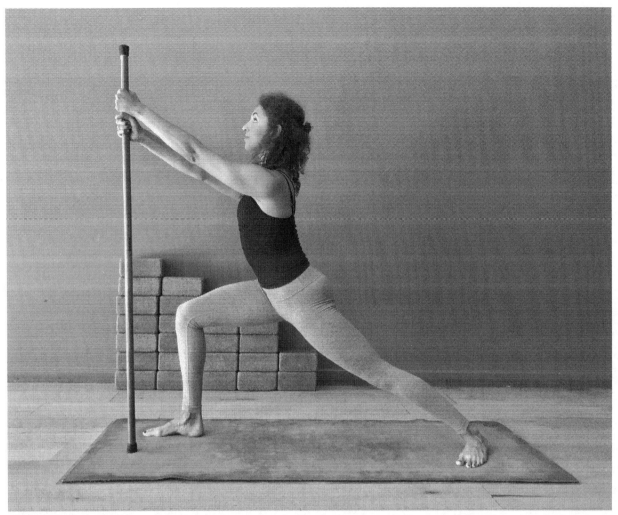

Side view

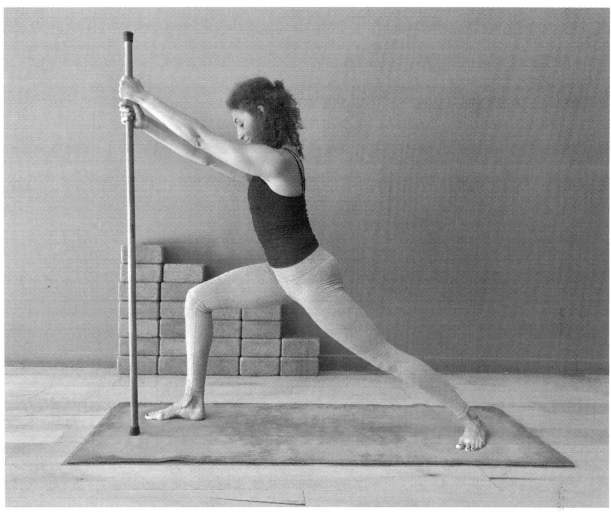

Side view

Warrior II

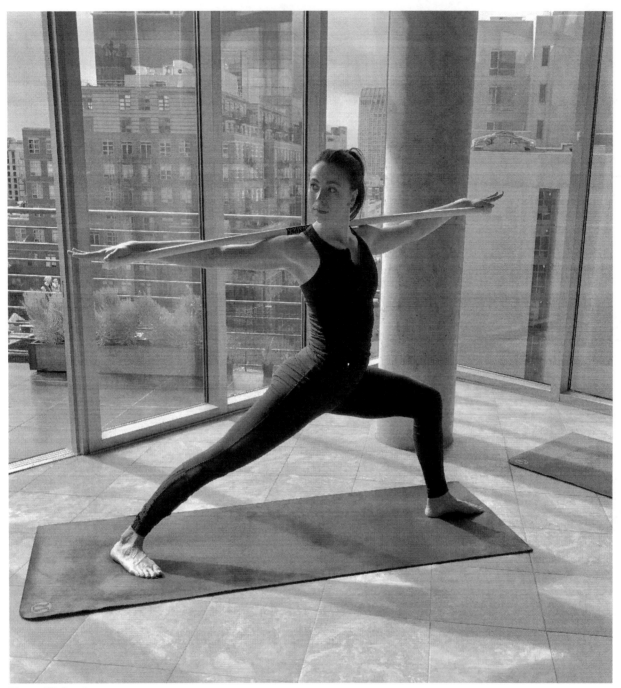

Rear Side view

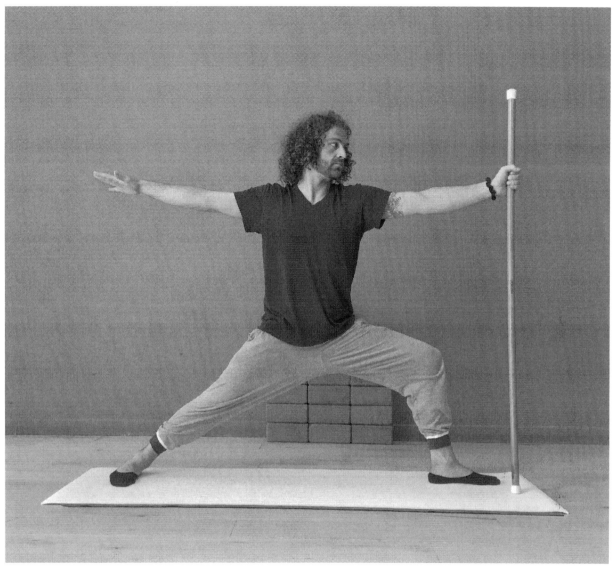

Side view

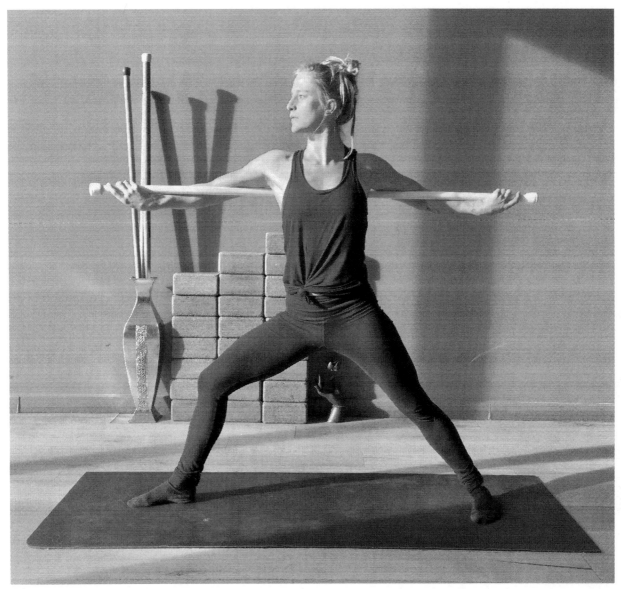
Front view

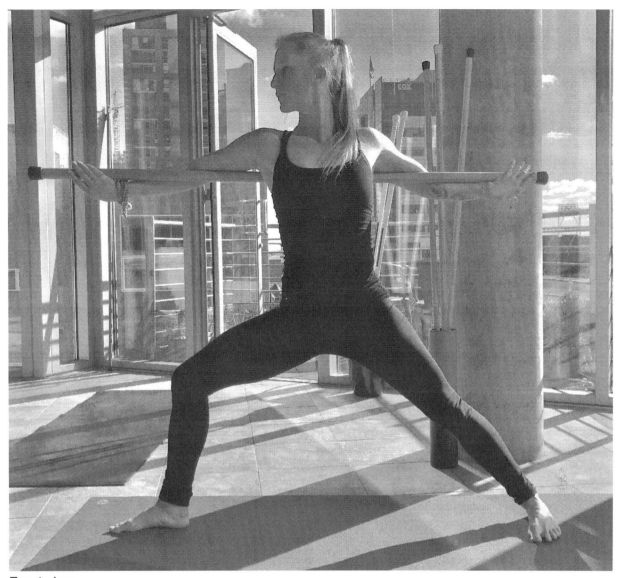

Front view

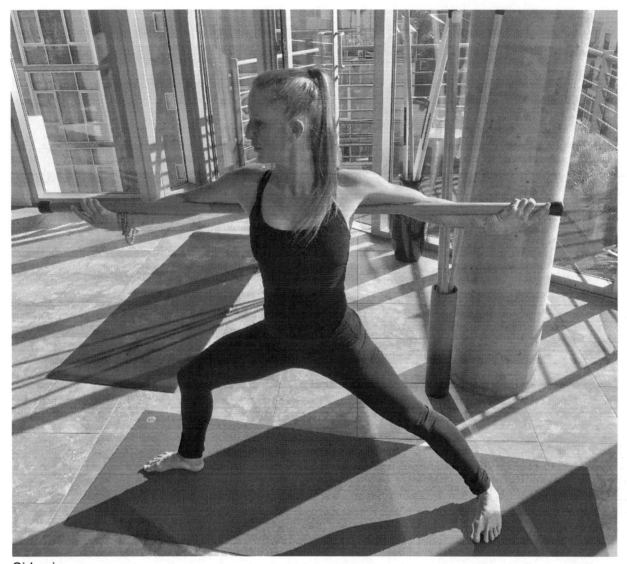
Side view

Warrior III

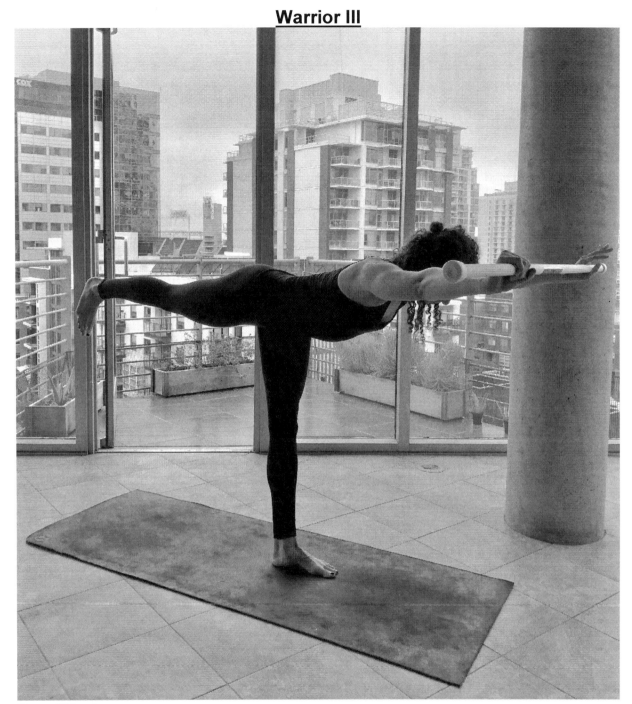

Front Side view

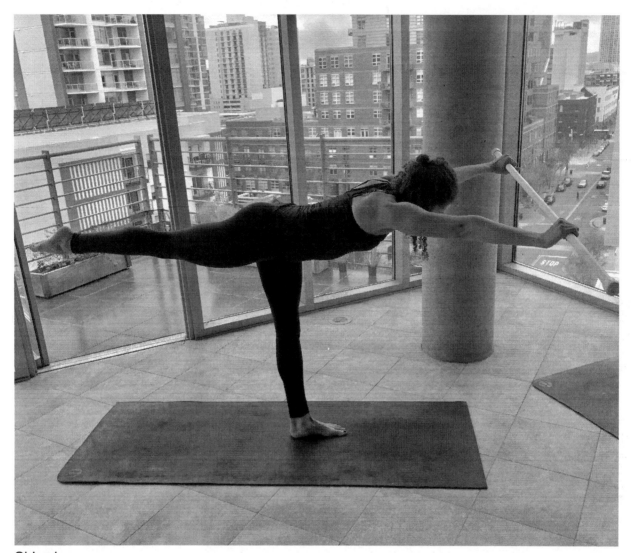

Side view

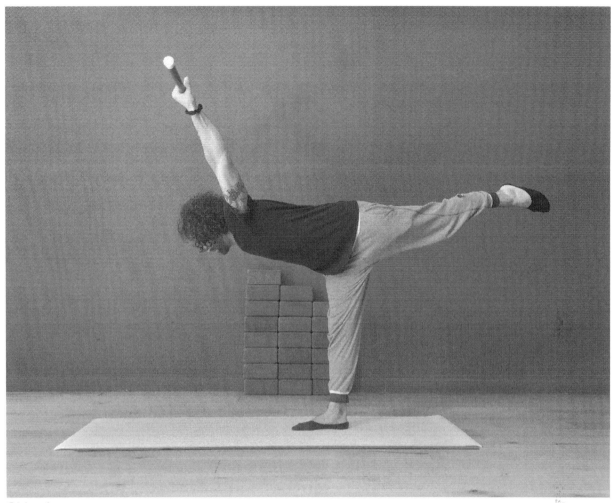

Side view

__Wavelength__

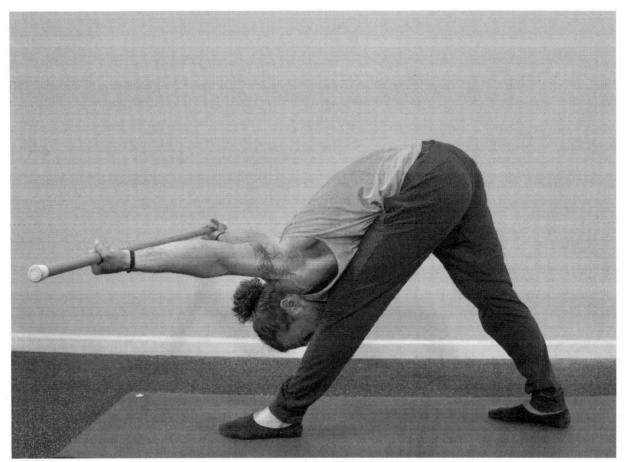
Side view

Wheel prep

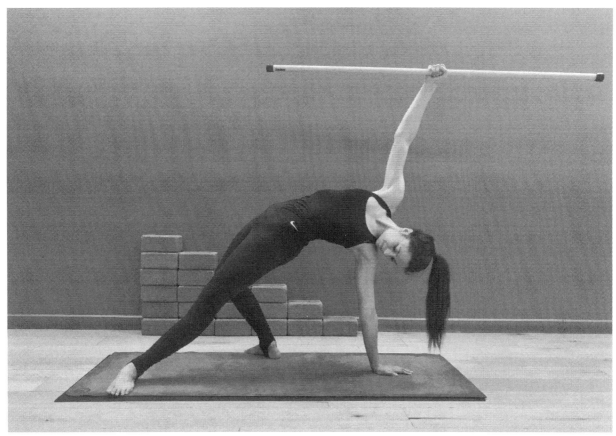
Side View

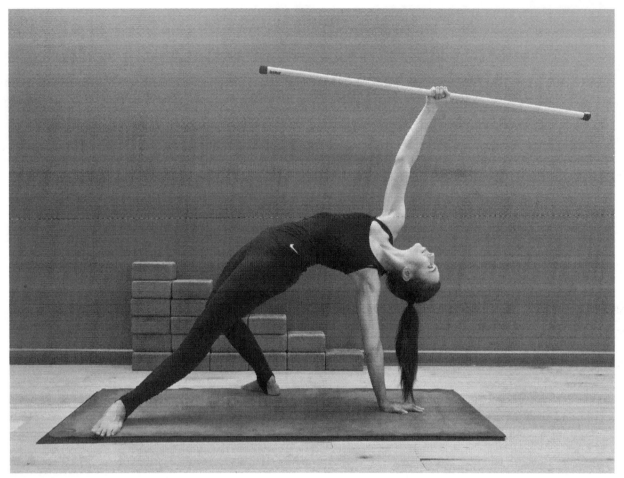
Side View

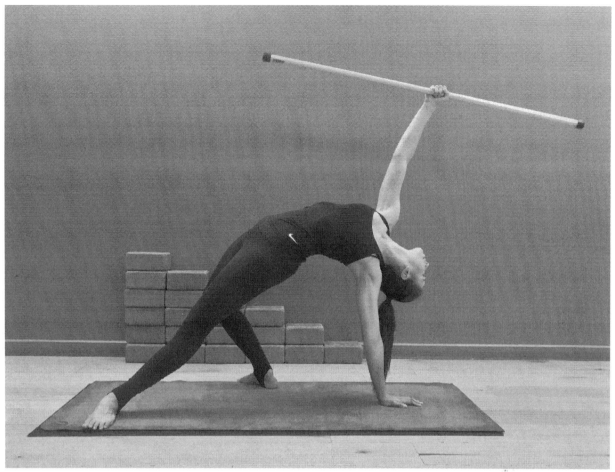
Side View

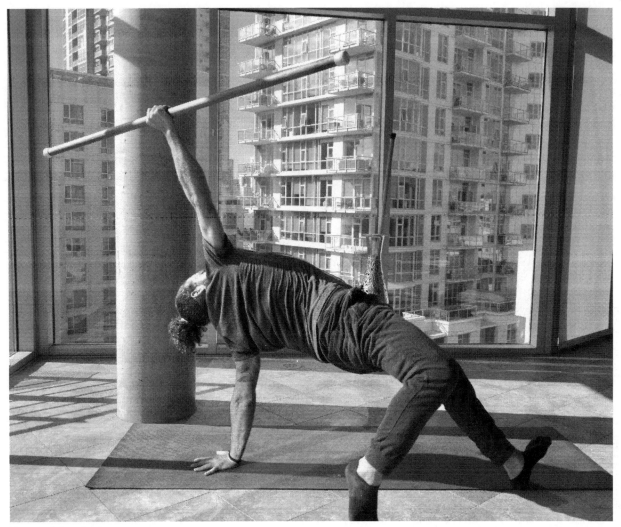
Rear side view

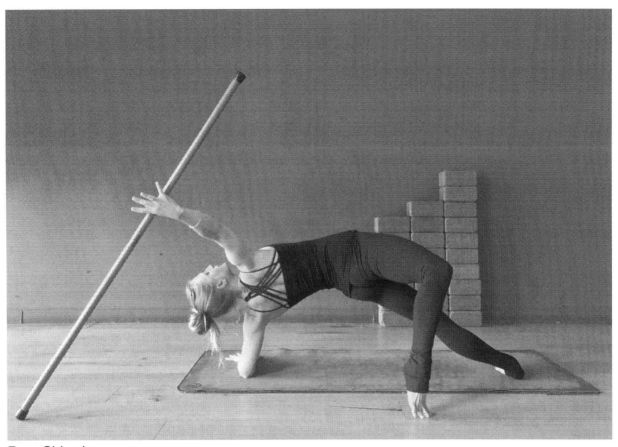

Rear Side view

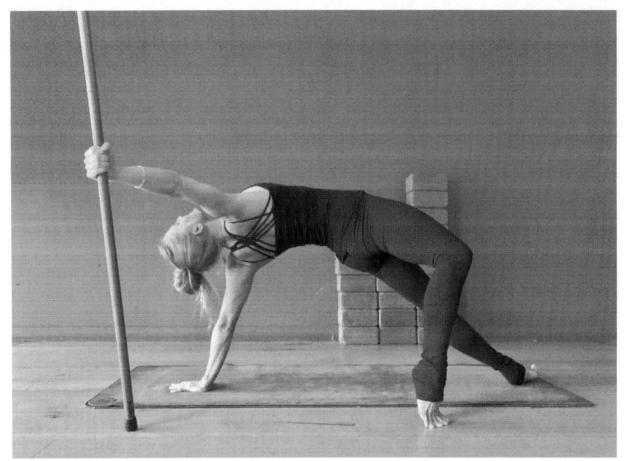

Rear Side view

402

Wind

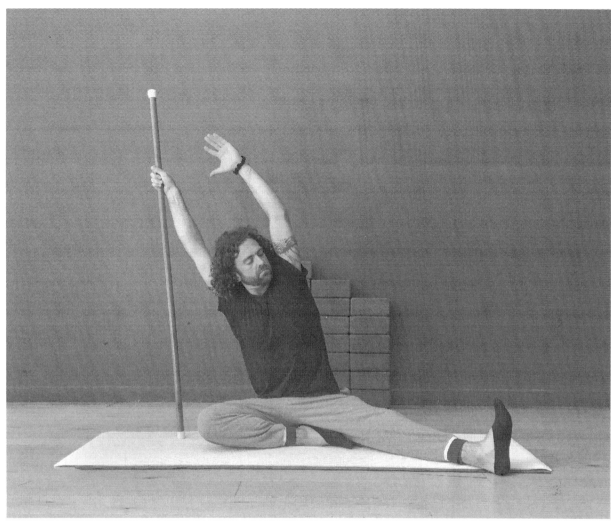

Front view

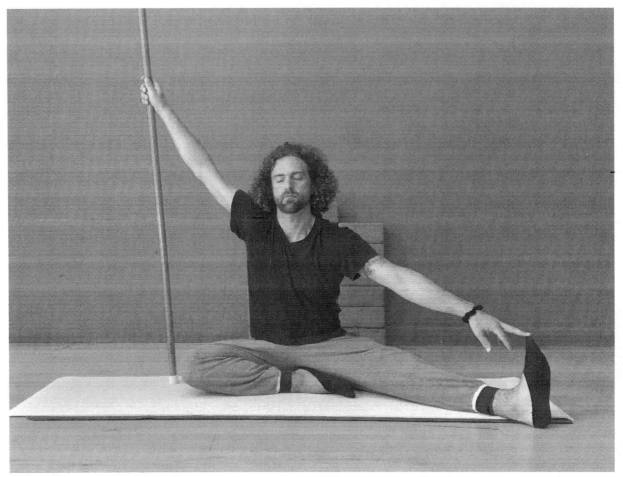

Front view

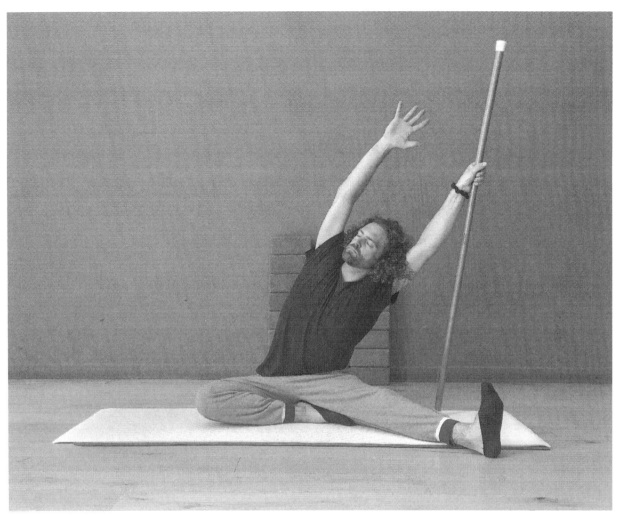

Front view

Wise Man

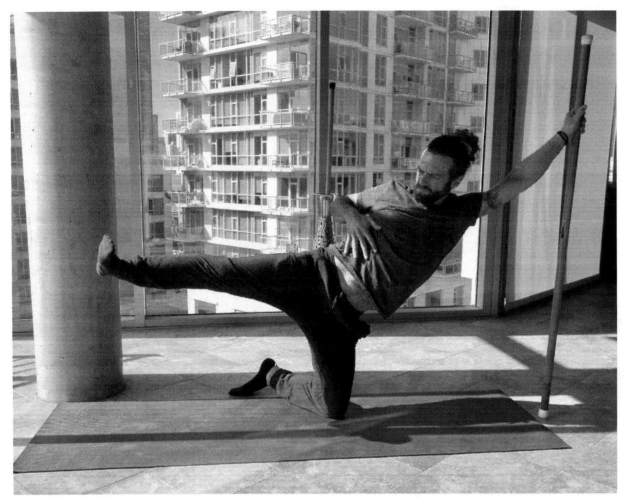

Front View

Wolverine

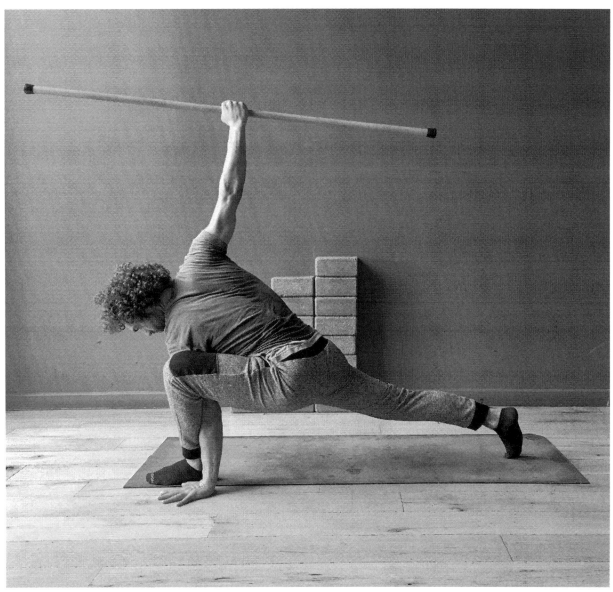

Side view

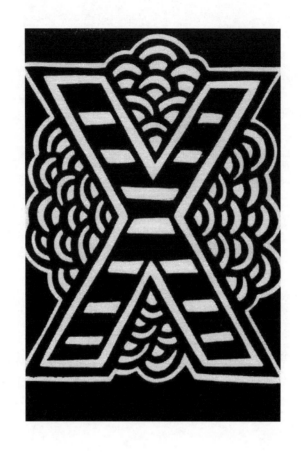

X-Ray

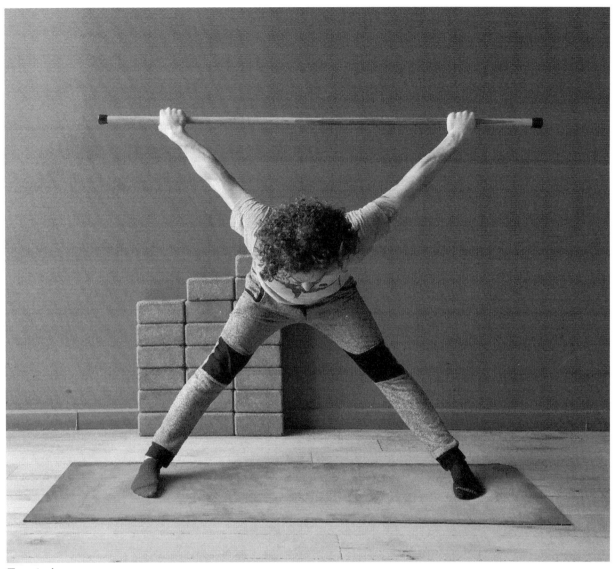

Front view

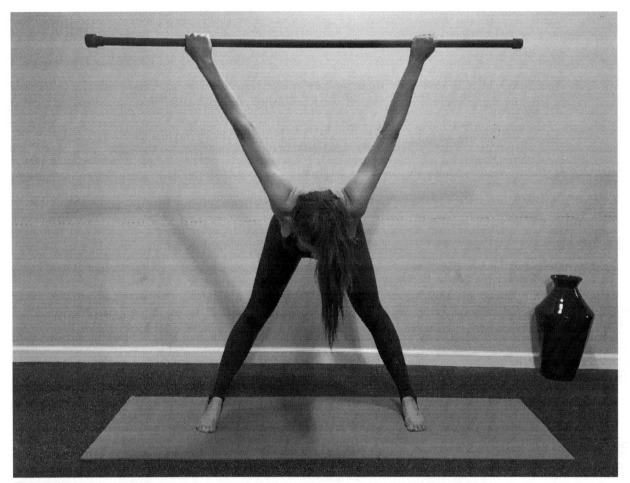

Front view

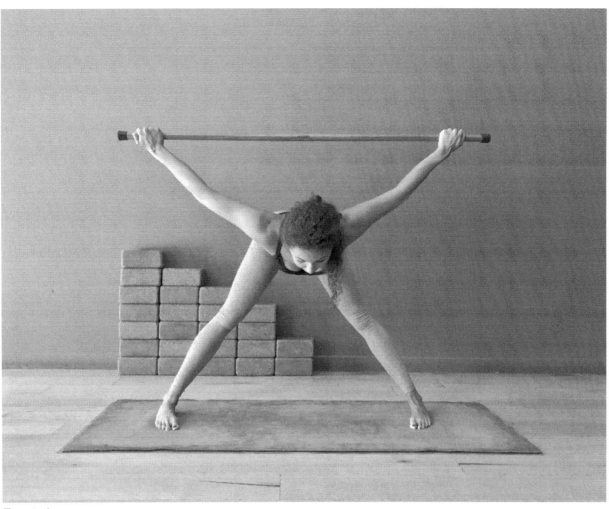

Front view

Xena Warrior

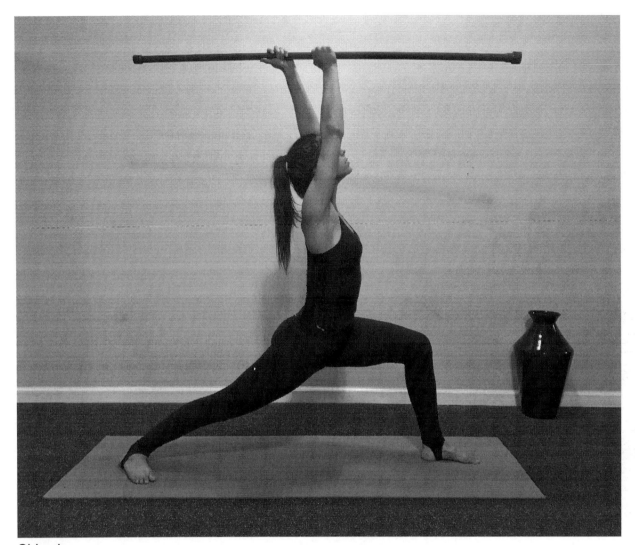
Side view

Xenopus

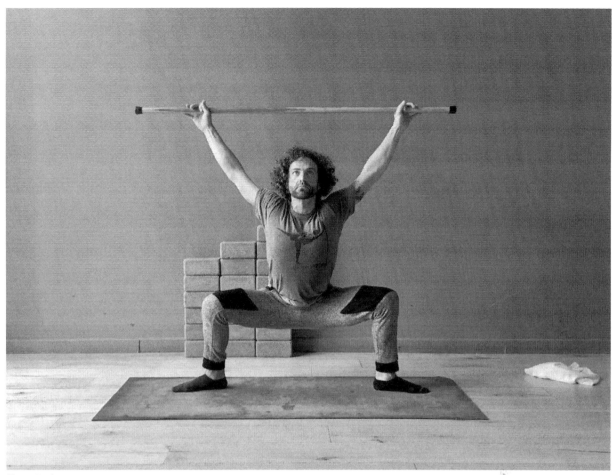

Front view

Xian (Flat Noodle)

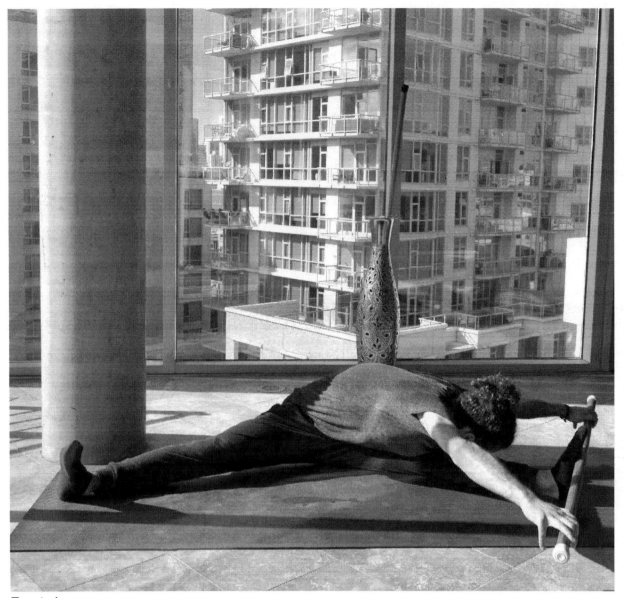

Front view

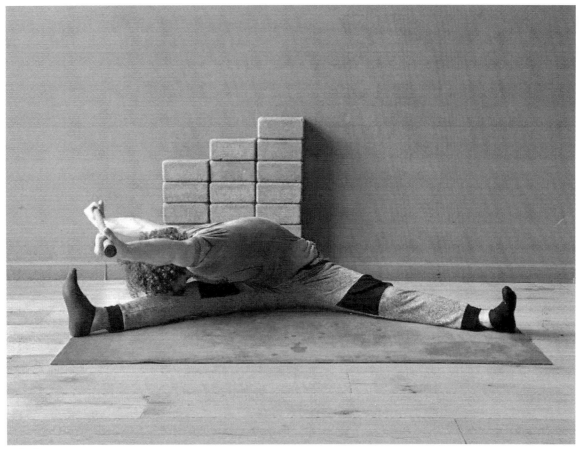

Front view

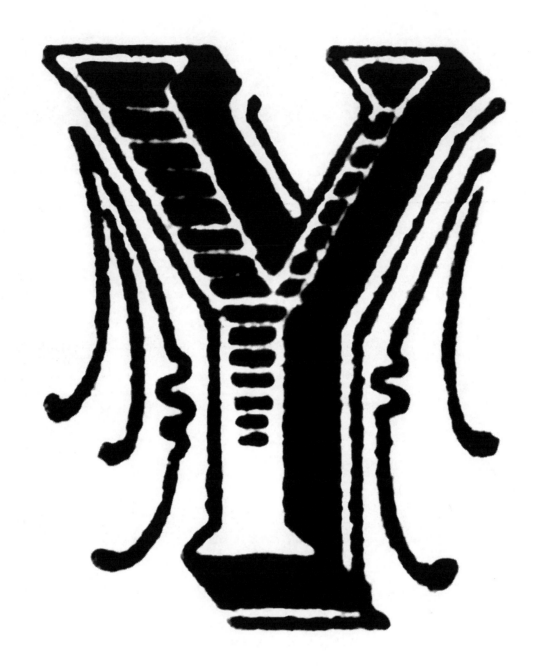

Yin Fold

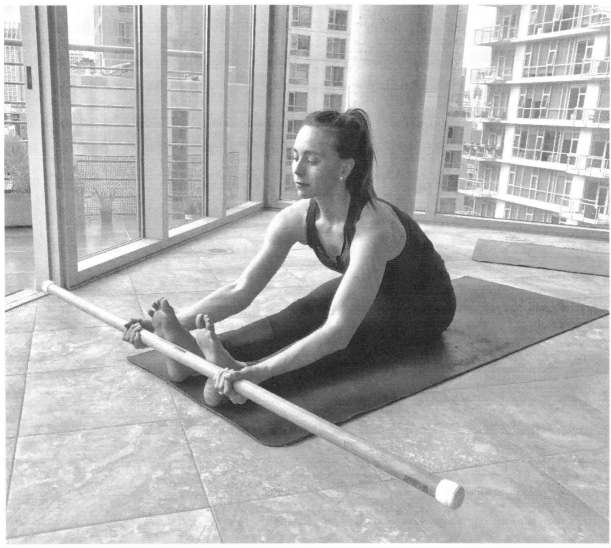
Front Side view

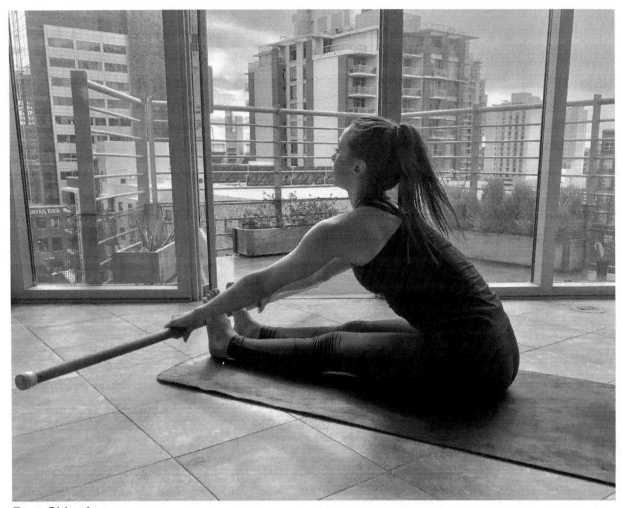

Rear Side view

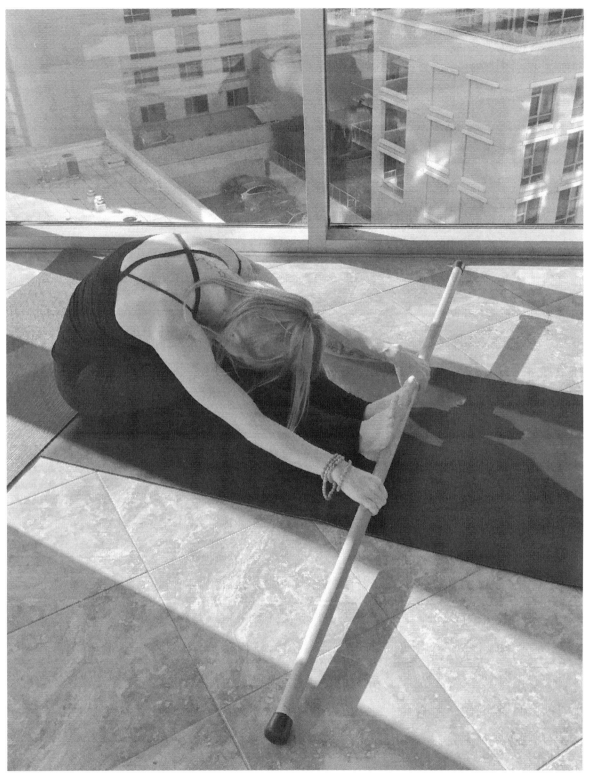

Side view

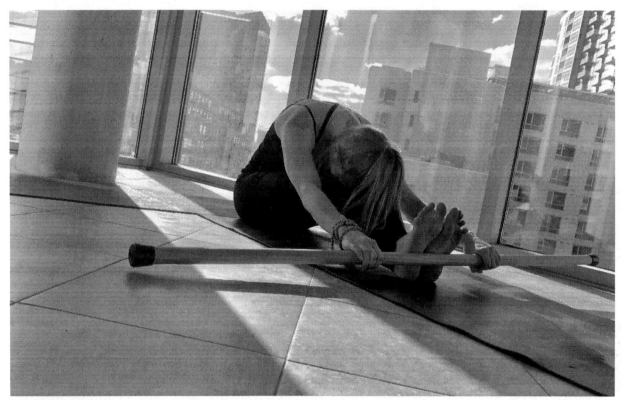
Front Side view

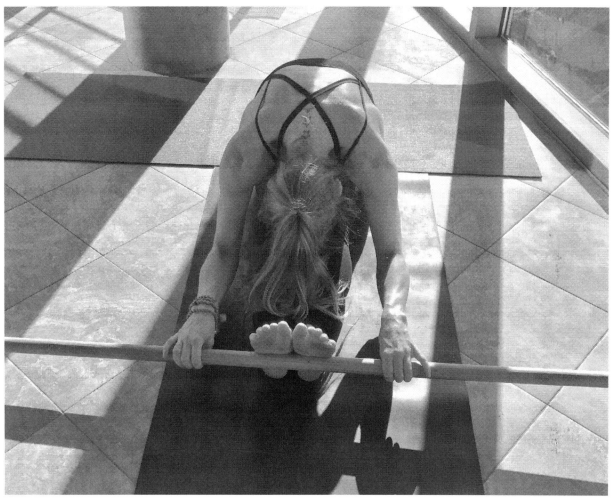
Front view

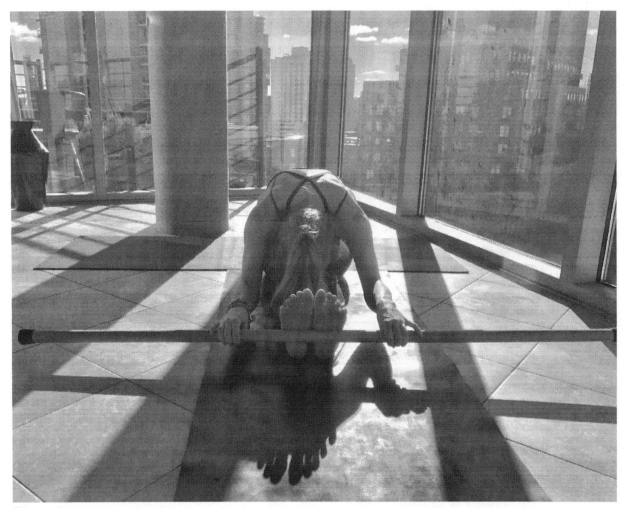

Front view

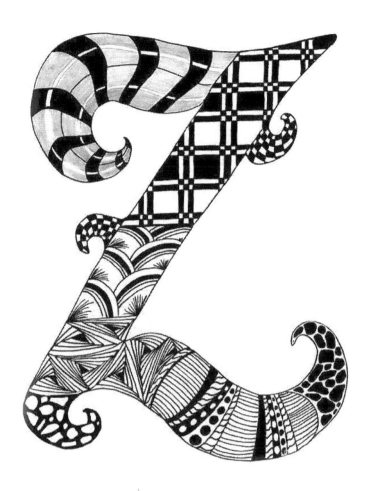

Zeus

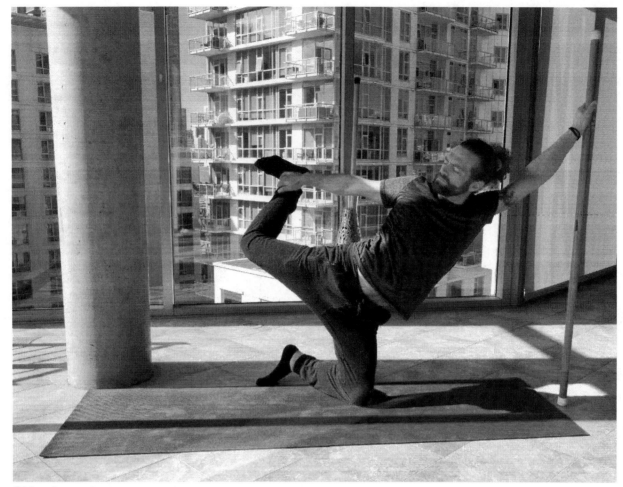
Side view

Zodiac

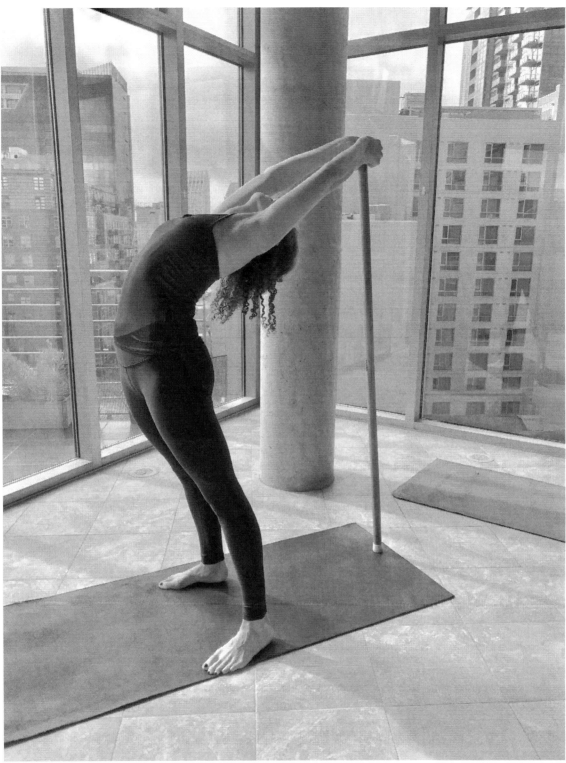

Front Side view

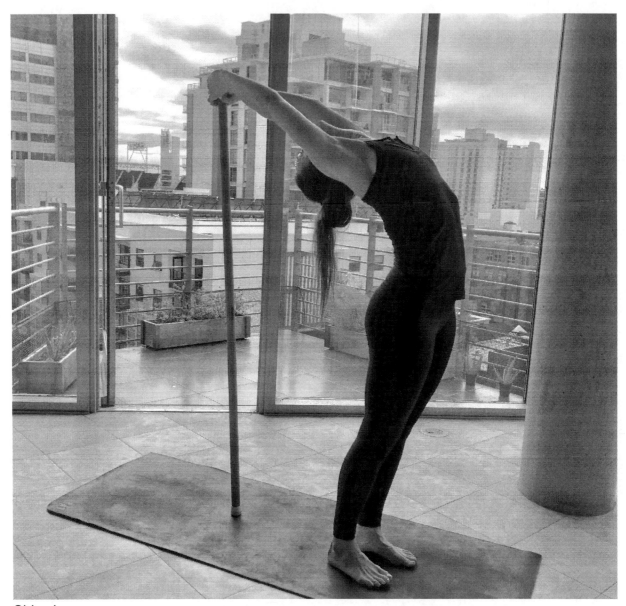

Side view

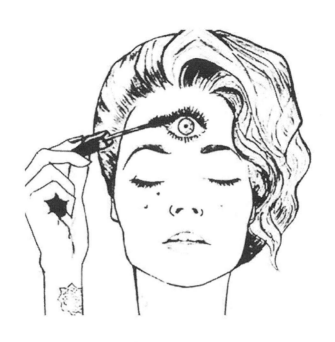

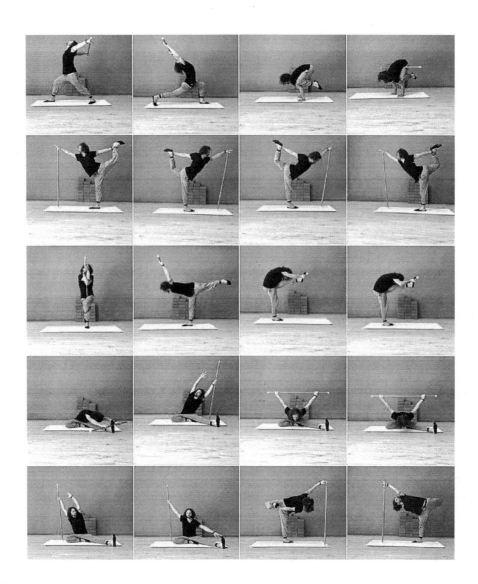

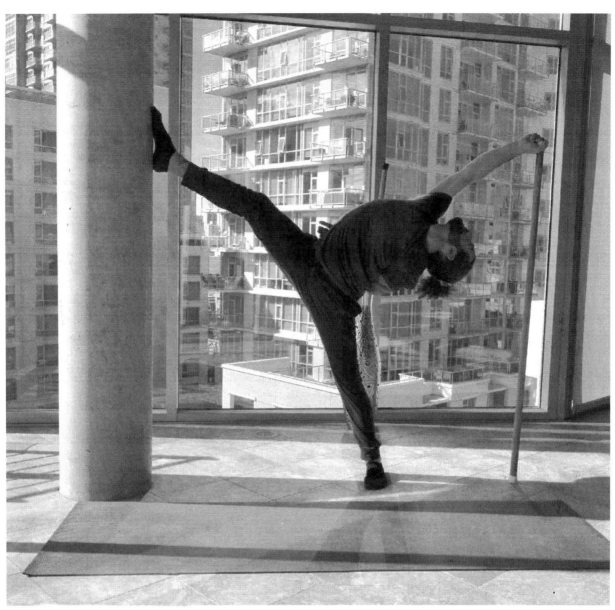

Front Side view

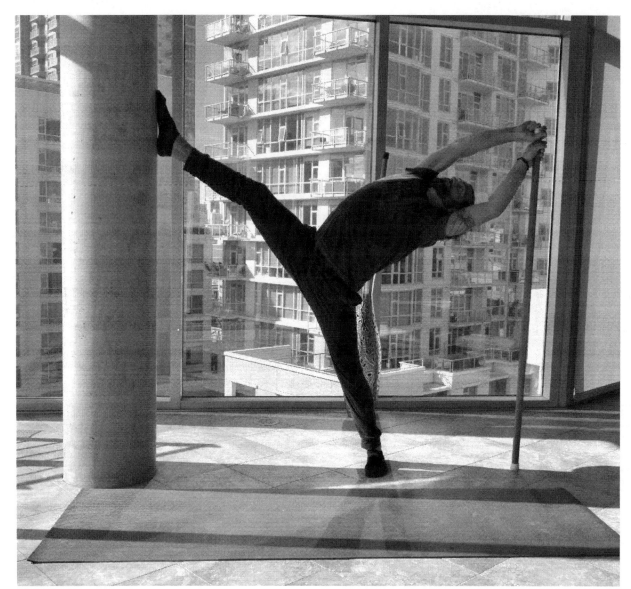

Front Side view

Index
Where multiple terms exist to describe a single pose, the alternative is given in parentheses.

A

Acceptance (Standing Forward Bend) 2,3
Albatross (Bound Prayer-Twist Lunge) 4,5,6,7
Angelfish (Fish out of Water) 8,9,10
Archer 11,12
Arm up the Wall 13,14,15
Asian Elephant (Low Lunge Prayer-Twist) 16,17
Aurora (Pistol Squat) 18
Axis (Seated Wide-Leg Halfway Lift) 19,20,21,22,23,24,25

B

Baby Crow 27,28,29
Balancing Half Moon (Great Wall) 151,152,153,154
Balancing Half Moon Reverse Foot Catch (Challenging) 58,59,60
Balancing Half Moon Variation (Super Moon) 350,351,352,353,354
Balancing Stick (Dhurva) 82,83,84,85
Ballerina 30
Barracuda (Locust) 31
Bharadvaja's Twist (Nature) 253
Bind & Balance (Bound Shiva Squat) 32
Birds of Paradise 33,34,35,36
Black Moon (Supported Candy Cane) 37,38
Bliss on Tap (Boat Tilted Head back) 39
Bloom & Prosper 40
Boat 41,42,43
Boat Arm-Twist (Solar Flare) 334
Boat Tilted Head back (Bliss on Tap) 39
Bound Extended Side Angle (Love is Binding) 225,226,227,228
Bound Prayer-Twist Lunge (Albatross) 4,5,6,7
Bound Shiva Squat (Bind & Balance) 32
Bound Standing Splits (Giraffe) 141
Bridge 44,45,46,
Butterfly (Flying Squirrel, Bound Angle) 126,127

C

Camel 48,49,50,51,52
Capricorn (Single-Arm High Lunge) 53,54

Chair 55,56,57
Chair Twist (Eskimo) 103,104,105,106,107
Chair Variation (Ostrich) 275,276
Challenging (Balancing Half Moon Reverse Foot Catch) 58,59,60
Champion (Dancing Shiva, Arm-Lift) 61
Child's Pose 62
Cobra (Up Dog) 380
Comet (Seated Half-Pigeon Solstice Arms) 63
Cow Lips (Pulsar) 291,292,293,294
Crescent (High Lunge Crescent) 64,65,66
Crane (Crow) 67,68,69
Crow (Crane) 67,68,69

D

Dancers 71,72,73,74,75
Dancing Shiva Arm-Lift (Champion) 61
Daring (Supported Reverse Dancers) 76,77
Deep Pockets (Half Pigeon Backbend) 78
DeJa Vu (Extended Hand-to-big toe) 79,80,81
Dhurva (Balancing Stick) 82,83,84,85
Dhurva Lama 86
Double Comet (Extended Balancing Half Moon) 87,88,89
Dreamer 90
Duck (Single-Legged Floor Bow) 91

E

Eagle 93,94,95
Earth (Wide-Legged Seated Forward Bend) 96,97
Eclipse (Revolved Standing Pyramid) 98,99
Eel 100

Elephant (Supported Balancing Half Moon) 101
Elevate 102
Eskimo (Chair Twist) 103,104,105,106,107
Evolve 108
Evolved Star 109
Exalted Warrior (Freedom) 131,132,132,133,134
Extended Balancing Half Moon (Double Comet) 87,88,89
Extended Hand-to-big toe (DeJa Vu) 79,80,81
Extended Hand-to-big toe (Libra) 213,214,215,216
Extended Side Angle 110,111,112,113
Extended Side Angle Variation (Impala) 184,185
Extended Standing Backbend (Zodiac) 425,426
Extended Triangle (Triangle) 366,367,368,369

F

Falcon (Revolved-Twist High Lunge) 115,116
Figure 4 Bridge (Umbra) 375
Firefly 117
Fire 118,119
Fire Log 120
Fish 121
Fish out of Water (Angelfish) 8,9,10
Flamingo 122,123,124
Floor Bow (Open Heart) 267,268,269,270,271
Flying Pigeon 125
Flying Squirrel (Butterfly, Bound Angle) 126,127
Folded Chair Variation (Pistol) 282,283
Folded Chair Variation (Sponge) 339
Forearm Side Plank 128,129,130
Freedom (Exalted Warrior) 131,132,133,134
Full Moon (Standing Side Bend) 135,136
Full Superman (Magnetic Field) 236

G

Garland (Horse, Frog) 178,179
Gate 138,139
Gemini (Wide-Legged Half Lift Arm Twist) 140
Giraffe (Bound Standing Splits) 141

Glacier (Side Lunge) 142,143
Goat (High Lunge Stretch) 144,145,146
Golden (One-Legged King Pigeon) 147,148,149
Grasshopper (Not So Easy) 256
Gratitude (Standing Hand-to-big toe Prep) 150
Great Wall (Balancing Half Moon) 151,152,153,154
Gypsy (One-Legged Bridge variation) 155
Gypsy Soul (One-Legged Bridge) 156,157

H

Half-Bound Horse (Nova) 257,258,259,260
Halfway Lift (Standing Half Forward Bend) 159
Halfway Lift Variation (Power) 288,289,290
Half Moon 160,161
Half Pigeon Backbend (Deep Pockets) 78
Half Splits 162,163,164,165,166
Happy Baby 167,168,169,170,171
Harry Potter 172
Heron (Kangaroo) 199
High Lunge 173,174,175,176,177
High Lunge Backbend (Inferno) 191
High Lunge Crescent (Crescent) 64,65,66
High Lunge Crescent Backbend (Queen L) 297,298,299,300
High Lunge Open Arm-Twist (Javelin) 194
High Lunge Stretch (Goat) 144,145,146
High Sprinter's Lunge (Sprinter) 338
Horse (Frog, Garland) 178,179
Horse Side-Bend (Red Giant) 304,305,306,307
Horse Variation (Xenopus) 413
Humble Gypsy 180,181
Humble Warrior 182

I

Impala (Extended Side Angle Variation) 184,185
Inclination 186,187
Indian Elephant (Revolved Triangle) 188,189,190
Inferno (High Lunge Backbend) 191
Intelligent 192
Intense Side Stretch (Teacher) 356,357

J

Javelin (High Lunge Open Arm-Twist) 194
Juice (Seated Arm-Twist) 195,196
Juno (Wide-Legged Forward Bend) 197

K

Kangaroo (Heron) 199
King Crab 200
King P (King Pigeon) 201,202,203,204,205
King Pigeon (King P.) 201,202,203,204,205
Kiss 206
Komodo D (One-Legged Head-to-knee Seated Forward Bend) 207,208,209

L

Ladybird 211
Lame Duck 212
Libra (Extended Hand-to-big toe) 213,214,215,216
Limb (Seated Revolved Head-to-Knee) 217,218,219,220

Llama 221,222,223,224
Locust (Barracuda) 31
Locust (Loveseat) 229,230,231
Locust Variation (Scorpio) 325,326,327
Love is Binding (Bound Extended Side Angle) 225,226,227,228
Loveseat (Locust) 229,230,231
Low Chair Squat (Porcupine) 287
Low Lunge 232,233,234
Low Lunge Open-Arm-Twist (Radial) 303
Low Lunge Open-Arm-Twist (Tsunami) 372,373
Low Lunge Prayer-Twist (Asian Elephant) 16,17

M

Magnetic Field (Full Superman) 236
Magnetic Pole 237
Meridian 238
Meteor (Supported Balancing Half Moon) 239,240,241,242
Miracle 243,244,245,246
Miracle Belt 247,248
Monkey 249
Mountain (Upward Salute) 250

N

Namaste 252
Nature (Bharadvaja's Twist) 253
Noah's Ark 254
Non Resistance (Splits Fold) 255
Not So Easy (Grasshopper) 256
Nova (Half-Bound Horse) 257,258,259,260
Number 4 261

O

Olympic 263,264,265
One-Legged Bridge (Gypsy Soul) 156,157
One-Legged Bridge Variation (Gypsy) 155
One-Legged Floor Bow (Duck) 91
One-Legged Head-to-knee Seated Forward Bend (Komodo D) 207,208,209
One-Legged King Pigeon (Golden) 147,148,149
Open Cluster 266
Open Heart (Floor Bow) 267,268,269,270,271
Opposition (Supported Candy Cane) 272,273
Orchid (Reverse Birds of Paradise) 274,275
Ostriche (Chair Variation) 276,277

P

Patience 279
Pigeon 280,281
Pistol (Folded Chair Variation) 282,283
Pistol Squat (Aurora) 18
Plow 284,285,286
Porcupine (Low Chair Squat) 287
Power (Halfway Lift Variation) 288,289,290
Pulsar (Cow Lips) 291,292,293,294
Pyramid 295
Pyramid (Wavelength) 396

Q

Queen L (High Lunge Crescent Backbend) 297,298,299,300
Quick 301

R

Radial (Low Lunge Open-Arm-Twist) 303
Red Giant (Horse Side-Bend) 304,305,306,307

Reverse Birds of Paradise (Orchid) 274,275
Reverse Dancers (Unicorn) 376,377,378,379
Reverse Triangle 308,309,310,311,312,313,314
Reverse Warrior 315,316,317
Revolved Bound Standing Splits (Sagittarius) 323,324
Revolved Side Angle (Trojan) 370,371
Revolved Standing Pyramid (Eclipse) 98,99
Revolved Triangle (Indian Elephant) 188,189,190
Revolved-Twist High Lunge (Falcon) 115,116
Risky (Splits) 318,319,320,321

S

Sagittarius (Revolved Bound Standing Splits) 323,324
Scorpio (Locust Variation) 325,326,327
Seahorse 328,329
Seated Arm-Twist (Juice) 195,196
Seated Forward Fold (Yin Fold) 417,418,419,420,421,422
Seated Half-Pigeon Solstice Arms (Comet) 63
Seated Revolved Head-to-Knee (Limb) 217,218,219,220
Seated Single-Leg Forehead-to-Knee (Volcano) 382,383
Seated Wide-Leg Half Lift (Axis) 19,20,21,22,23,24,25
Shoulder Stand 330
Side Lunge (Glacier) 142,143
Side Plank 331
Side Star 332
Single-Arm High Lunge (Capricorn) 53,54
Single-Legged Floor Bow (Duck) 91
Smile 333
Solar Flare (Boat Arm-Twist) 334
Solstice 335
Spectrum 336,337
Splits (Risky) 316,317,318,319
Splits Fold (Non Resistance) 255

Sprinter (High Sprinter's Lunge) 338
Sponge (Folded Chair Variation) 339
SSLFK (Standing Separate-Leg Forehead-to-Knee) 340,341,342,343,344
Standing Forward Bend (Acceptance) 2,3
Standing Half Forward Bend (Half Lift) 159
Standing Hand-to-big toe Prep (Gratitude) 150
Standing Separate-Leg Forehead-to-Knee (SSLFK) 340,341,342,343,344
Standing Side Bend (Full Moon) 135,136

Standing Splits 345,346,347
Standing Wide-Legged Halfway Lift (X-Ray) 409,410,411
Sunspot 348,349
Super Moon (Balancing Half Moon Variation) 350,351,352,353,354
Supported Balancing Half Moon (Elephant) 101
Supported Balancing Half Moon (Meteor) 239,240,241,242
Supported Balancing Half Moon (Wise Man) 406
Supported Candy Cane (Black Moon) 272,273
Supported Candy Cane (Opposition) 37,38
Supported Dancers (Zeus) 424
Supported Reverse Dancers (Daring) 76,77

T

Teacher (Intense Side Stretch) 356,357
Terrestrial 358
Tiptoe 359
Tree 360,361,362
Tree Frog 363
Tree Top 364,365
Triangle (Extended Triangle) 366,367,368,369
Trojan (Revolved Side Angle) 370,371
Tsunami (Low Lunge Open-Arm-Twist) 372,373

U

Umbra (Figure 4 Bridge) 375
Unicorn (Reverse Dancers) 376,377,378,379
Up Dog (Cobra) 380
Upward Salute (Mountain) 250

V

Volcano (Seated Single-Leg Forehead-to-Knee) 382,383

W

Warrior I 385,386,387
Warrior II 388,389,390,391,392
Warrior III 393,394,395
Wavelength (Pyramid) 396
Wheel Prep (Wild Thing) 397,398,399,400,401,402
Wide-Legged Forward Bend (Juno) 197
Wide-Legged Half Lift Arm-Twist (Gemini) 140
Wide-Legged Seated Forward Bend (Earth) 96,97

Wild Thing (Wheel Prep) 397,398,399,400,401,402
Wind 403,404,405
Wise Man (Supported Balancing Half Moon) 406
Wolverine 407

X

X-Ray (Standing Wide-Legged Halfway Lift) 409,410,411
Xena Warrior 412
Xenopus (Horse Variation) 413
Xian 414,415

Y

Yin Fold (Seated Forward Fold) 417,418,419,420,421,422

Z

Zeus (Supported Dancers) 424
Zodiac (Extended Standing Backbend) 425,426

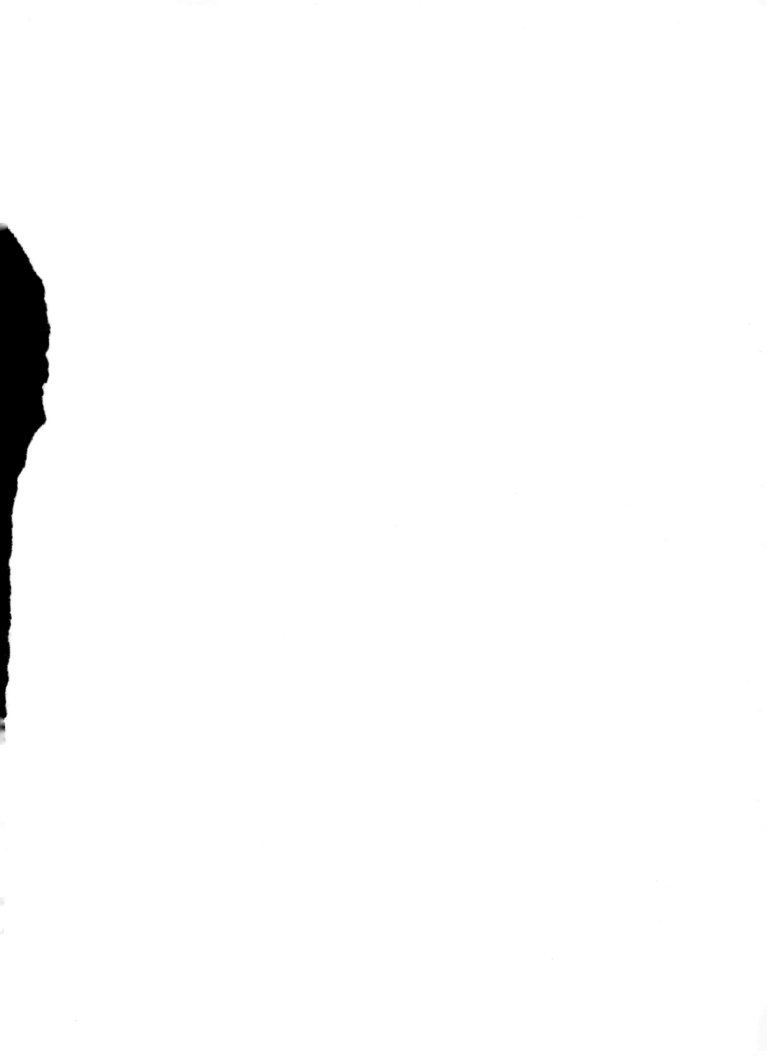

Made in the USA
San Bernardino, CA
17 May 2017